Heart to Heart:

A Plunge

into

the Everyday Life

of a

Cardiology nursing

assistant

MARTIN STERLING

« *Working in cardiology is a bit like being an orchestra conductor: you make sure that every beat is*

in rhythm, and you pray that no one decides to play their own score in the middle of the symphony! »

Table of contents

Chapter 2: Technical skills of the Cardiac Caregiver

Chapter 4: Prevention and Therapeutic Education in Cardiology

Chapter 5: Continuing Professional Development for Cardiology Nurses

Introduction

- **The crucial role of the cardiology orderly**
  - Importance in the medical team

The cardiology orderly occupies a central position in the medical team, playing an indispensable role that often goes beyond simple technical tasks. They are the direct link between the patient and other healthcare professionals, guaranteeing the continuity of care essential to the smooth running of the department. They are often the first to detect subtle signs of deterioration in a patient's state of health, thanks to their constant observation and in-depth knowledge of the behaviors and symptoms characteristic of heart disease.

Their role is not limited to carrying out tasks delegated by nurses or doctors. They actively contribute to clinical assessment, monitoring vital parameters, noting changes in the patient's general condition, and communicating these observations clearly and accurately to other team members. This vigilance helps to anticipate and prevent potential complications, which is crucial in such a sensitive environment as cardiology, where every minute can be decisive.

Caregivers also play a key role in managing the physical and emotional well-being of patients. Hygiene care, mobilization and daily accompaniment contribute not only to patient comfort, but also to recovery. The relationship of trust he establishes with patients and their families is often a determining factor in their adherence to treatment and their morale. This proximity enables them to act as empathetic intermediaries, passing on crucial information on the patient's emotional and psychological state to other team members, often as important as clinical data.

Cardiac orderlies are also distinguished by their ability to work under pressure, in emergency situations where every decision can have vital consequences. Their cool-headedness, expertise and speed of execution make them an essential player in critical interventions, such as cardiac arrest or hypertensive crises. He provides invaluable support to doctors and nurses, enabling them to concentrate on their specific tasks while ensuring optimum coordination of care.

Finally, the cardiology orderly helps to educate patients, informing them of the steps they need to take to manage their condition, reassuring them about upcoming procedures, and guiding them through the stages of their rehabilitation. This educational role is vital, as it prepares patients to become active players in their own health, promoting better compliance with treatment and reducing the risk of readmission.

o   Impact on patients

The caregiver's impact on cardiology patients is profound and multifaceted, affecting their physical, emotional and psychological well-being. In cardiology, where every moment can be critical and every detail counts, the caregiver plays an essential role in the patient experience, often beyond what is immediately visible.

From the moment a patient arrives, the caregiver is often the first person with whom he or she interacts, establishing an initial contact that can set the tone for the entire stay. With their reassuring attitude and empathetic approach, they help reduce the anxiety inherent in hospitalization, especially in a context as sensitive as that of heart disease. This ability to allay the patient's fears is crucial, as a more relaxed patient is more receptive to care and explanations, improving adherence to treatment and overall recovery.

The nursing auxiliary is also directly involved in the patient's physical comfort and well-being. He or she ensures that hygiene care is carried out gently, that the patient is properly mobilized to avoid complications such as bedsores, and that pain is effectively managed. Through their constant presence, they ensure that the patient's basic needs are met, often even before they express them. This daily support is particularly vital for cardiology patients, who may feel particularly vulnerable due to the severity of their condition.

On an emotional level, the caregiver's role is one of moral support, listening to the patient's worries and fears. He or she creates a space of trust where the patient feels safe to share anxieties, which can considerably lighten the mental burden of illness. This relationship of trust not only reinforces the patient's state of mind, but also provides valuable information about his or her feelings, symptoms and general comfort, which can be relayed to other members of the healthcare team.

The caregiver also has an impact on patient rehabilitation. After an operation or during the recovery phase, they are the ones who encourage patients to gradually resume their activities, take part in rehabilitation exercises, and adopt a lifestyle compatible with their heart condition. This day-to-day motivation, made up of small encouragements and thoughtful gestures, can make all the difference to the patient's recovery, giving him or her the strength to overcome physical and psychological obstacles.

Last but not least, the caregiver's impact also extends to supporting families. By explaining care, reassuring about procedures, and answering questions, they help relatives understand and adapt to the patient's situation. This creates a supportive environment where the patient feels surrounded not only by his or her family, but also by the medical team, reinforcing the patient's sense of security and well-being.

- **Why this book?**
  ◦ Objectives: Encourage, inform and support

The aims of a book dedicated to the cardiology orderly must be clear and ambitious: to encourage, inform and support. These three pillars are essential to meet the needs of students and novices in this specialty, offering them not only knowledge, but also the motivation and support they need to excel in their profession.

Above all, **encouragement** means recognizing the value of the caregiver's role and giving them the means to believe in their abilities. Working in cardiology can be demanding and at times taxing, both physically and emotionally. It is therefore crucial to remind caregivers of the importance of their mission, their impact on patients' lives, and the recognition they deserve within the healthcare team. Such encouragement involves highlighting daily successes, small victories that, when accumulated, make a big difference. It also means highlighting the specific skills developed in this field, showing how they contribute directly to the well-being and healing of patients. The aim is for every reader to feel inspired, strengthened in their commitment, and proud of their contribution.

Providing information is a fundamental objective, as cardiology is a complex field in which knowledge is rapidly evolving. A well-designed book should provide caregivers with all the information they need to understand heart disease, its associated treatments, and the specific care they need to provide. The aim is not simply to pass on technical data, but to make it accessible and relevant to their daily practice. Information must be accurate, up-to-date and adapted to the specific context of the caregiver's role. This includes not only medical knowledge, but also care protocols, technological innovations and specific approaches to managing critical situations. By being well-informed, caregivers gain confidence, efficiency and safety in their work.

Support is perhaps the most humane and essential goal. Accompanying means offering ongoing support through the challenges caregivers face in their daily work in cardiology. This book is intended to be a companion, ready to answer questions, dispel doubts and provide practical advice. The aim is to support not only learning, but also reflection on practices, stress management and professional development. Coaching must also include a psychological aspect, offering tools for managing the emotional, maintaining a positive attitude in the face of challenges, and finding a balance between the demands of the job and personal well-being. This holistic support is essential if caregivers are not only to survive in their working environment, but also to flourish and evolve.

○   How to use this book

This book has been designed to be a companion, a practical and accessible guide that every cardiac caregiver can use to train, improve and find support throughout their career. Its use must be intuitive, adapted to the varied needs of readers, whether students, novices or experienced professionals. The aim is for this book not simply to sit on a shelf, but to be consulted regularly, leafed through, annotated, and truly integrated into daily practice.

To get the most out of this book, it's important to approach it as a living resource. Rather than reading it in a linear fashion, chapter by chapter, it can be useful to use it according to the situations you encounter on a daily basis. If you're faced with a particular clinical case or a specific question, go straight to the relevant chapter or section. Each part has been designed to be self-contained, enabling quick and efficient consultation. For example, if you need to review the steps involved in a post-operative procedure or refresh your knowledge of vital parameter monitoring, you'll be able to access the relevant information easily.

This book is also a progressive learning tool. If you're just starting out or have recently joined a cardiology department, start with the introductory chapters, which will give you an overview of the department, the diseases you'll encounter, and the role you'll play. As you gain experience, you can deepen your knowledge by exploring the more technical sections, the case studies, or the chapters dedicated to technological innovations and emergency situations. This progression will enable you to consolidate your skills in a coherent way, reinforcing both your theoretical knowledge and your daily practice.

In addition to learning and applying knowledge, this book can also serve as a source of inspiration and reflection. The chapters dedicated to testimonials, field stories and ethical aspects offer enriching perspectives that can nourish your approach to the profession. By reading about the experiences of other caregivers, you can recognize yourself in their challenges, but also find ideas and advice for improving your own practice. What's more, these stories can help you maintain a strong connection with the human essence of your work, reminding you of the importance of empathy, communication and compassion in caring.

Finally, this book can be a valuable tool for self-assessment and ongoing professional development. Through the various sections, you'll be able to identify your strengths as well as areas where you'd like to improve. Feel free to use this book to plan your training objectives, to prepare discussions with colleagues or supervisors, or to reflect on your career development. It can also be used to support training sessions or discussion groups within your department, enabling you to share best practices and collectively improve the quality of care you provide.

Chapter 1

Understanding the Cardiology Department

The foundations of cardiology

○   Introduction to cardiovascular disease

Cardiovascular disease is one of the world's leading causes of morbidity and mortality, affecting millions of people every year. Understanding these diseases is essential for any healthcare professional working in cardiology, and even more so for nursing aides, who are on the front line in the care and monitoring of patients suffering from these pathologies. This introduction aims to provide an overview of the main cardiovascular diseases, their impact on health, and the importance of their management.

Cardiovascular disease covers a wide range of conditions affecting the heart and blood vessels. Among the most common are coronary artery disease, high blood pressure, heart failure, arrhythmias and heart valve disease. Each of these pathologies has specific characteristics, but they all share a common factor: they compromise the heart's ability to ensure efficient blood circulation, which can lead to serious, even fatal, complications if not properly managed.

Coronary artery disease, also known as ischemic heart disease, is one of the most common forms of cardiovascular disease. It is characterized by a narrowing or obstruction of the coronary arteries, which are responsible for supplying blood to the heart muscle. This narrowing is often due to the accumulation of atheromatous plaques, a mixture of fats, cholesterol and other substances that build up on the artery walls. When blood flow to the heart is reduced, this can lead to chest pain, known as angina pectoris, and in more serious cases, a myocardial infarction, or heart attack.

Hypertension, often dubbed the "silent killer", is another common cardiovascular disease. It is characterized by excessive blood pressure against artery walls, which can lead to a series of serious complications if left unchecked. Hypertension can damage the arteries, making the walls thicker and less flexible, increasing the risk of heart attacks, strokes and kidney failure. It is often asymptomatic, which means that many people are unaware they have it until complications arise.

Heart failure is another major pathology in the cardiovascular field. Unlike a heart attack, which is an acute event, heart failure is a chronic condition in which the heart is unable to pump enough blood to meet the body's needs. This can result from weakness of the heart muscle (systolic dysfunction) or an inability of the heart to fill properly (diastolic dysfunction). Patients with heart failure may experience symptoms such as fatigue, shortness of breath, and fluid accumulation in the lungs and extremities, requiring close monitoring and ongoing care.

Arrhythmias, or heart rhythm disorders, are another crucial aspect of cardiovascular disease. To function properly, the heart must beat at a regular rhythm. Arrhythmias occur when the electrical signals that regulate this rhythm are disturbed, causing the heart to beat too fast (tachycardia), too slow (bradycardia), or irregularly. Some arrhythmias can be benign, while others, such as atrial fibrillation or ventricular tachycardia, can be life-threatening and require immediate intervention.

Finally, heart valve diseases are conditions that affect the heart's valves, responsible for regulating blood flow through the various heart chambers. When the valves fail to function properly, blood flow can be disrupted, leading to symptoms such as shortness of breath, fatigue and edema. These conditions can be congenital or acquired, and their treatment can range from medical management to reconstructive surgery or valve replacement.

Understanding these cardiovascular diseases is essential for cardiology caregivers, as it enables them to intervene in a more informed and effective way in the day-to-day care of patients. Knowing the symptoms, risks and treatments associated with each pathology helps not only to better monitor and support patients, but also to anticipate potential complications and actively contribute to their prevention.

○ The main conditions encountered in cardiology: angina pectoris, heart attack, heart failure, etc.

In cardiology, certain conditions are frequently encountered and require special attention from healthcare professionals, including orderlies. Although these conditions vary in terms of severity and treatment, they all share a common denominator: they affect the heart and blood vessels, jeopardizing patients' overall health. Among these conditions, angina pectoris, myocardial infarction and heart failure are among the most common, but it's also crucial to consider other conditions such as arrhythmias and heart valve disease.

Angina pectoris, also known as angina, is a condition characterized by chest pain due to a temporary reduction in blood supply to the heart muscle. This ischemia is usually caused by a partial obstruction of the coronary arteries, often due to atherosclerosis, an accumulation of fatty plaques on the arterial walls. Patients often describe the pain as a feeling of pressure or tightness, sometimes radiating to the left arm, neck or jaw. Angina pectoris can be stable, occurring with physical effort or stress, or unstable, occurring unpredictably and potentially heralding a myocardial infarction. In all cases, prompt treatment is essential to relieve symptoms and prevent serious complications.

Myocardial infarction, commonly known as heart attack, is a medical emergency in which one or more coronary arteries become completely blocked, preventing oxygen supply to part of the heart muscle. This prolonged interruption of blood flow leads to necrosis of heart tissue, irreversible damage that can seriously compromise cardiac function. Symptoms of a heart attack include intense, prolonged chest pain, often described as a crushing weight, accompanied by sweating, nausea, breathing difficulties, and sometimes loss of consciousness. Rapid intervention is crucial to restore blood flow, usually by thrombolysis or angioplasty, and limit damage to the heart. The caregiver's role in quickly recognizing the signs of a heart attack and immediately alerting other team members is vital to the patient's survival.

Heart failure is a chronic condition in which the heart is unable to pump enough blood to meet the body's needs. It may result from weakness of the heart muscle (systolic insufficiency) or from the heart's inability to fill properly (diastolic insufficiency). Underlying causes can be multiple, including ischemic heart disease, valvular heart disease, hypertension and cardiomyopathy. Symptoms of heart failure include dyspnea (shortness of breath), excessive fatigue, peripheral edema (swelling of the legs and feet), and sometimes pleural effusions or ascites. Management of this condition requires a multidisciplinary approach, including rigorous monitoring of vital parameters, administration of medication, and dietary advice to reduce fluid retention. The caregiver plays a key role in ensuring patient comfort, monitoring the evolution of symptoms, and assisting in the implementation of therapeutic measures.

Cardiac arrhythmias are heart rhythm disorders that can manifest themselves as beats that are too fast (tachycardia), too slow (bradycardia), or irregular (atrial fibrillation). Some arrhythmias may be benign and require only regular monitoring, while others, such as ventricular fibrillation, are potentially life-threatening and require immediate intervention. Symptoms vary from mild palpitations to dizziness, chest pain or syncope (loss of consciousness). The caregiver must be able to detect the signs of an arrhythmia, quickly alert nurses and doctors, and assist in resuscitation procedures if necessary.

Heart valve disease affects the valves that regulate blood flow through the heart's chambers. Valves can be stenotic (narrowed), preventing blood from flowing freely, or insufficient, failing to close properly and allowing blood to flow backwards. These conditions may be congenital or acquired, often following an infection such as rheumatic fever. Symptoms include fatigue, shortness of breath, palpitations and peripheral swelling. Management can range from regular monitoring to surgery to replace or repair the failing valve.

These main conditions encountered in cardiology require rigorous management and continuous monitoring. For the nursing auxiliary, understanding these diseases and their clinical manifestations is essential not only to provide appropriate care, but also to play a proactive role in preventing complications and improving patients' quality of life. Working in close collaboration with the rest of the medical team, the orderly contributes directly to the overall care and well-being of patients, which is at the heart of his or her mission in cardiology.

○   Developments in cardiology techniques and care

The evolution of techniques and care in cardiology is a field marked by rapid and continuous progress, which has transformed the way heart disease is diagnosed, treated and managed. These advances have not only improved patient survival rates, but have also profoundly changed the daily lives of healthcare professionals, including orderlies, whose role has adapted to the new demands and opportunities offered by these innovations.

Over the decades, cardiology has benefited from a series of technological revolutions that have enabled heart disease to be diagnosed earlier and treated in a more targeted, less invasive way. One of the most significant advances has been the development of medical imaging, notably echocardiography, computed tomography (CT) and magnetic resonance imaging (MRI). These tools enable detailed visualization of the heart and blood vessels, facilitating precise diagnosis of various pathologies such as congenital heart disease, heart valve abnormalities and coronary artery disease. For the caregiver, these technologies have introduced new tasks linked to preparing patients for these examinations, managing the data collected, and accompanying patients who are often anxious about these procedures.

Interventional cardiology is another field that has undergone spectacular development. The introduction of angioplasty, a technique for dilating blocked coronary arteries using a balloon and stents, has revolutionized the treatment of myocardial infarction and angina pectoris. This technique, which often avoids the need for open-heart surgery, has considerably reduced the mortality associated with heart attacks. It has also shortened recovery times and improved patients' quality of life. For caregivers, this means greater involvement in post-operative care, monitoring vital signs, and educating patients about caring for themselves at home after surgery.

Advances in pharmacological treatment have also transformed cardiology care. The development of drugs such as beta-blockers, ACE inhibitors, angiotensin II receptor antagonists and anticoagulants has radically changed the management of heart disease. These treatments provide better control of hypertension, prevent recurrence of heart attacks, and manage heart failure more effectively. The introduction of new classes of drugs, such as PCSK9 inhibitors for cholesterol reduction, continues to expand the available therapeutic options. For the caregiver, this means constant vigilance in administering medication, monitoring side effects, and educating patients on the importance of therapeutic compliance.

Surgical techniques have also evolved significantly, notably with the rise of minimally invasive surgery and robotic surgery. These techniques enable complex procedures, such as heart valve repair or replacement, to be carried out with smaller incisions, less pain, and shorter recovery times. For the caregiver, this translates into specific post-operative care, where wound monitoring, pain management, and support for early mobilization of patients play a crucial role in the healing process.

Telemedicine and remote patient monitoring are other fast-growing fields, particularly for patients suffering from heart failure or heart rhythm disorders. Thanks to home monitoring devices, patients can measure their blood pressure, heart rate or other vital parameters and transmit this data to their care team in real time. This enables more proactive and personalized care management, with rapid adjustments to treatments if necessary. For the caregiver, this introduces new responsibilities in terms of training patients to use these devices, collecting and interpreting data, and coordinating with other members of the healthcare team.

The evolution of techniques and care in cardiology is not limited to technological and medical aspects; it also encompasses a more holistic, patient-centered approach. Cardiac rehabilitation, which combines supervised exercise programs, dietary advice and psychological support, has become a key element in the management of post-infarction and other heart diseases. This comprehensive approach aims to reduce the risk of recurrence, improve quality of life, and promote rapid and safe reintegration into daily life. The caregiver plays an essential role in this phase, motivating patients, monitoring their progress, and supporting them in adopting new lifestyle habits.

The organization of a cardiology department

o   Structure of a cardiology department: intensive care units, conventional hospitalization, outpatient consultations

The structure of a cardiology department is designed to provide an efficient, specialized response to the varied needs of patients suffering from cardiovascular disease. This organization is based on segmentation into a number of distinct units, each with a specific role in managing patients at different stages of their care. The main components of this structure include intensive care units, conventional hospitalization and outpatient consultations. Each unit plays a complementary role, ensuring complete and continuous care for patients, from the moment they enter the department through to their post-hospital follow-up.

Cardiac Intensive Care Units (CICUs) are highly specialized areas where critically ill patients or those at high risk of complications are cared for. These units are equipped with advanced continuous monitoring technologies, enabling vital parameters such as heart rate, blood pressure, oxygen saturation and heart rhythm to be monitored in real time. Patients admitted to intensive care units are often those who have suffered a myocardial infarction, acute heart failure, or severe arrhythmia requiring urgent intervention. The nursing staff in these units, comprising doctors, nurses and specially trained orderlies, work closely together to provide rapid, intensive care. The caregiver, in particular, plays a key role in monitoring patients, administering daily care, and assisting with complex procedures, thus contributing directly to the stabilization and recovery of critically ill patients.

Conventional cardiology hospitalization is for patients who require continuous medical monitoring, but whose condition does not require the intensive care provided in the ICU. Patients admitted to these units are often those recovering from cardiac surgery, angioplasty, or an exacerbation of their chronic heart disease, such as heart failure. This part of the department is structured to enable close follow-up, while offering patients a more stable and less intensive environment than intensive care. Rooms are equipped with appropriate monitoring devices, and nursing staff ensure regular monitoring of vital parameters, administration of treatments, and daily assessment of patients' clinical condition. In this context, the nursing auxiliary is essential for basic care such as hygiene, mobilization and nutrition, as well as for psychological support for patients in the recovery phase. They also play an important role in educating patients and their families, preparing them to return home and manage their condition independently.

Cardiology outpatient clinics are the third major component of the department's structure. They are intended for patients requiring regular follow-up, diagnostic assessments or specialized outpatient consultations. Outpatient clinics are the main point of contact for many chronic patients, such as those suffering from hypertension, stable coronary disease or valvular heart disease, as well as for post-operative or post-interventional follow-up. Outpatient consultations are used to assess disease progression, adjust treatments and plan future interventions. The caregiver's role in this unit is mainly focused on preparing patients for examinations (such as electrocardiograms or echocardiograms), assisting with consultations, and coordinating care with other departments. The orderly may also be involved in taking measurements such as blood pressure or weight, essential data for patient assessment.

- The various players in the department: doctors, nurses, care assistants, technicians, etc.

The Cardiology Department functions thanks to the close, coordinated collaboration of a number of players, each contributing their specific expertise to ensure optimum patient care. This multidisciplinary team is made up of doctors, nurses, orderlies, technicians and other healthcare professionals, all united by a common goal: to provide the best possible care for patients suffering from cardiovascular disease. Complementary roles and effective communication between these different players are essential to the smooth running of the department and the quality of the care provided.

Cardiologists play a central role in the department. They are responsible for the diagnosis, treatment and follow-up of patients. Cardiologists are involved at several levels: outpatient consultations, hospitalization management, intensive care interventions, and the performance of medical procedures such as angioplasties, echocardiography and electrophysiology. Their role is to make a precise diagnosis based on clinical and paraclinical examinations, to define a therapeutic strategy adapted to each patient, and to supervise the implementation of care. As orchestrators of treatment, cardiologists work closely with other team members to ensure that each patient receives coherent, coordinated care, while taking into account individual specificities.

Nurses, meanwhile, play a crucial role in the day-to-day administration of care. They are the guarantors of continuity of care, ensuring that medical prescriptions are followed to the letter and that patients' needs are met in real time. Nurses monitor vital parameters, manage drug therapy, provide technical care such as dressings, infusions and catheter care, and provide therapeutic education for patients. In intensive care, their role is even more critical, as they are responsible for constantly monitoring the most unstable patients, intervening rapidly in the event of a deterioration in clinical condition, and supporting patients and their families through these difficult times. They are also key contacts for the nursing assistants, guiding them in their daily tasks and ensuring smooth coordination of care.

Nurses' aides are an essential part of the care team, providing the basic care that is vital to a patient's well-being. Their role goes far beyond hygiene and comfort; they are the eyes and ears of the team, often the first to detect a subtle change in a patient's condition. Caregivers are responsible for grooming, assisting with mobility, taking meals, and providing psychological support to patients, thus contributing to their physical and moral recovery. Their constant presence at patients' bedsides enables them to develop a relationship of trust, listen to patients' concerns, and relay this valuable information to the nursing team. In emergency situations, they are also involved in first aid, preparing patients for interventions, and assisting nurses with specific procedures.

Cardiology technicians provide essential technical expertise, particularly in the performance and interpretation of paraclinical examinations. They are responsible for managing monitoring equipment, electrocardiograms, echocardiograms and other diagnostic tools. Their role is crucial in ensuring the quality and reliability of the medical data on which doctors base their therapeutic decisions. In addition to carrying out these examinations, technicians are responsible for the maintenance and smooth running of the equipment, ensuring that the healthcare team always has the resources it needs for accurate diagnosis and effective monitoring.

Other professionals, such as physiotherapists, dieticians and psychologists, also work in the cardiology department, contributing their specific expertise to the overall care of patients. **Physiotherapists** play a key role in cardiac rehabilitation, helping patients to regain their mobility and resume appropriate physical activity after surgery or hospitalization. **Dieticians** are essential in advising patients on a diet suited to their cardiovascular condition, helping to prevent relapses and improve quality of life. **Psychologists**, meanwhile, provide indispensable support to help patients overcome the anxiety, stress and emotional challenges associated with heart disease.

Finally, the efficiency of the cardiology department also relies on the work of the **medical secretaries** and **administrative staff**, who manage the logistical aspects, coordinate appointments, ensure communication between the various departments, and make sure that the patient's journey is as smooth as possible, from admission to discharge.

        ◦   Workflow and interprofessional collaboration

Workflow in a cardiology department is a complex and dynamic process, based on close, well-coordinated interprofessional collaboration. Each member of the team, whether doctor, nurse, orderly, technician or other healthcare professional, plays a specific role, but it is their ability to work together smoothly and harmoniously that ensures efficient and safe patient care. This inter-professional collaboration is the very foundation of the service's success, where communication, coordination and cooperation are essential at every stage of the care process.

The workflow often begins with patient admission, where each professional has a well-defined task. **Doctors** make an initial diagnosis, order the necessary tests, and draw up a care plan. **Nurses**, for their part, take charge of implementing this plan, ensuring that treatments are administered correctly and that the patient's immediate needs are met. **Nurses' aides** play a crucial role at this stage, welcoming the patient, making him or her comfortable, and carrying out basic care, while remaining alert to signs of distress or discomfort. Their constant presence with the patient ensures constant monitoring, facilitating early detection of any complications.

Interprofessional collaboration is also evident at **medical staffs**, regular meetings where the healthcare team comes together to discuss patient cases, exchange information, and adjust treatment plans as the clinical situation evolves. These meetings are essential to ensure that all team members share a common vision and are aligned on care objectives. The opinions of everyone, from doctors to technicians, are taken into account, as each perspective brings a more complete understanding of the patient's situation. These moments of exchange also serve to strengthen team cohesion, by valuing each member's contribution and fostering a climate of mutual trust.

In the day-to-day running of the department, the workflow is punctuated by a series of interdependent activities. **Medical procedures such as** angioplasty, electrophysiology or echocardiography are performed by cardiologists, often assisted by specialized technicians. **Nurses** prepare patients for these procedures, provide post-intervention monitoring, and coordinate care with other departments where necessary. **Nurses**, for their part, are involved in logistical preparation, accompanying patients to the procedure rooms, and re-installing them in the units after the procedure. Each stage is marked by constant communication, where information on the patient's condition, specific needs, and actions to be taken are shared clearly and precisely.

Interprofessional collaboration is also crucial in emergency situations, where speed of execution and coordination are vital. When a patient presents with a sudden deterioration in condition, such as a heart attack or serious arrhythmia, the entire team must react in perfect synchronization. **Doctors** make rapid decisions on the treatment to be administered, **nurses** prepare and administer drugs or set up resuscitation devices, while **orderlies** assist by providing the necessary equipment, ensuring the patient's safety, and helping to perform emergency procedures. Every second counts, and it's the team's ability to work together seamlessly that can make the difference between life and death.

Apart from emergency situations, the workflow also includes **preparation for return home** or transfer to other services, where inter-professional collaboration continues to play a key role. **Nurses and orderlies** ensure that the patient and family fully understand the instructions for home management, the treatments to be followed, and the warning signs to watch out for. **Medical secretaries and administrative staff coordinate** the logistical aspects, such as scheduling follow-up appointments, supplying medication, and managing medical records. Here again, clear communication and good coordination are essential to avoid errors and ensure a smooth transition.

Chapter 2

Technical skills of the Cardiology Orderly

Monitoring specific vital parameters

- Blood pressure monitoring: Methods, frequency and interpretation of results

Blood pressure monitoring is an essential task in cardiology, as it enables the detection and close monitoring of blood pressure variations, which can be valuable indicators of a patient's state of health. This is all the more crucial in a department where patients are often at risk of serious cardiovascular complications, such as myocardial infarction, heart failure or stroke. Effective management of these patients relies on rigorous blood pressure monitoring, including precise methods, appropriate frequency of assessment, and correct interpretation of results.

The methods used to measure blood pressure are varied, but the aim remains the same: to obtain reliable, reproducible values that reflect the patient's hemodynamic state. The most commonly used method is sphygmomanometer measurement, which can be manual (with an inflatable cuff and stethoscope) or automated (with an electronic device). The choice of method depends on the clinical context, but in all cases it is essential to follow a standardized protocol to minimize measurement errors. Blood pressure is generally measured at upper arm level, with the patient in a sitting or lying position, after a few minutes' rest to avoid the influence of stress or recent physical activity. The caregiver, who is often in charge of this task, must ensure that the cuff is correctly positioned at heart level and that the patient is relaxed, as these factors can greatly influence the results.

The frequency of blood pressure monitoring depends on the patient's clinical condition and the context in which he or she is being cared for. For a patient hospitalized in an intensive care unit, blood pressure may be measured continuously using an invasive or non-invasive monitoring device, enabling real-time monitoring of blood pressure variations. In a less acute setting, such as conventional inpatient or outpatient care, the frequency of measurements may vary from several times a day to once a week, depending on the patient's stability and therapeutic goals. For example, in a hypertensive patient on treatment, closer monitoring may be required to adjust medication and prevent complications. Caregivers must be vigilant as to the regularity of measurements and the consistency of the technique used, as the reliability of the data depends on it.

Interpretation of blood pressure monitoring **results** is a critical aspect of care, as it guides clinical decisions. Normal blood pressure values are generally considered to be below 140/90 mmHg, although these thresholds may vary according to age, comorbidities and disease-specific recommendations. High blood pressure, or hypertension, may indicate an increased risk of cardiovascular complications, requiring prompt intervention to avoid organ damage. Conversely, low blood pressure, or hypotension, can signal hypoperfusion of vital organs, which is of particular concern in critically ill patients. The caregiver plays a key role in the initial interpretation of these results, immediately alerting the nursing team to any abnormal values or significant variations from previous measurements.

It is also important to take into account **factors that may influence results**, such as stress, pain, recent medication use, or even technical errors during measurement. The caregiver must be able to identify these factors and communicate them to the rest of the team for a full clinical assessment. For example, a sudden rise in blood pressure may be due to an episode of acute pain or the patient's anxiety, rather than a real deterioration in his or her cardiovascular condition.

○   Heart rate and rhythm monitoring

Monitoring heart rate and rhythm is a fundamental component of cardiology care, helping to detect and manage abnormalities in heart function that can have serious consequences for patients. Careful, continuous monitoring of these parameters is essential, not only to diagnose cardiac disorders, but also to monitor the effectiveness of treatments and anticipate complications. The caregiver's role in this process is crucial, as he or she is often in

41

the front line of observing, measuring and reporting variations in heart rate and rhythm, thus contributing directly to the overall management of patients.

Heart rate, the number of beats per minute, is a key indicator of a patient's hemodynamic status. A normal resting heart rate is generally between 60 and 100 beats per minute. Deviations from this norm may indicate clinical conditions requiring special attention. **Tachycardia**, defined as a heart rate above 100 beats per minute, may be a sign of a physiological response to stress, pain or infection, but it can also reveal more serious cardiac disorders, such as heart failure, supraventricular arrhythmia or myocardial infarction. Conversely, **bradycardia**, characterized by a heart rate below 60 beats per minute, may be normal in some patients, such as athletes, but can also be a sign of atrioventricular block, hypothermia or drug intoxication.

Heart rhythm refers to the regularity of the heartbeat. A normal heart rhythm, known as sinus rhythm, is regular, with a constant interval between beats. **Arrhythmias**, or irregularities in heart rhythm, can vary in severity, from simple, often benign extrasystoles, to potentially life-threatening conditions such as ventricular fibrillation or ventricular tachycardia. Early identification of these arrhythmias is crucial to prevent severe complications such as cardiac arrest or stroke. The caregiver, in his or her role of continuous monitoring, is in a position to spot these anomalies early, thanks to the use of monitoring devices, auscultation or pulse palpation.

Methods for monitoring heart rate and rhythm are varied and depend on the patient's clinical condition. Monitoring can be performed non-invasively, by palpation of the radial or carotid pulse, or using an electrocardiogram (ECG), which records the heart's electrical activity and enables detailed rhythm analysis. In intensive care units or for high-risk patients, continuous monitoring is often used, with electrodes attached to the patient's chest and connected to a monitor that displays heart rate and rhythm in real time. This allows instant detection of any deviation from normal, and rapid reaction in the event of an emergency.

Interpretation of the results is a key step, as it guides clinical decisions. An abnormally high or low heart rate, or an irregular rhythm, must be assessed in the overall context of the patient's condition. For example, tachycardia may require further evaluation to determine the cause, whether dehydration, anxiety or an underlying cardiac disorder. Similarly, persistent bradycardia may require further investigation, particularly if accompanied by symptoms such as dizziness or fainting. The caregiver plays an essential role in immediately reporting any abnormality to the rest of the nursing team, enabling rapid and appropriate management.

As part of post-operative follow-up or in patients undergoing rehabilitation, regular monitoring of heart rate and rhythm is also crucial for assessing response to treatment and adjusting care if necessary. For example, after a procedure such as stenting or cardiac surgery, careful monitoring can help detect early complications such as persistent tachycardia or new arrhythmias. The caregiver, through his or her constant observation and knowledge of the patient, is often the first to notice these subtle but significant changes.

Finally, **educating patients** about monitoring their own heart rate and the warning signs to watch out for is an important aspect of the caregiver's role. Teaching patients how to take their pulse, recognize the symptoms of palpitations or irregular heartbeats, and know when to seek medical attention, is crucial to their empowerment and to preventing long-term complications.

- ○ Using and monitoring monitoring devices

The use and monitoring of monitoring devices are fundamental elements in the management of cardiology patients. These devices enable continuous monitoring of vital patient parameters such as heart rate, blood pressure, oxygen saturation and other critical indicators, providing a real-time overview of the patient's hemodynamic status. The accuracy and reliability of these data are essential for detecting early abnormalities, preventing serious complications, and adapting treatments accordingly. The role of the caregiver in the use and monitoring of these devices is crucial, as it ensures not only that the devices function correctly, but also that the data can be rapidly interpreted for appropriate intervention.

Installing the monitoring devices is a key first step, where the caregiver must ensure that each sensor is correctly positioned and attached to the patient. Electrodes for cardiac monitoring must be placed in precise locations on the chest to ensure accurate heart rate readings. Similarly, the blood pressure cuff must be positioned at heart level and correctly adjusted to avoid measurement errors. For oxygen saturation monitoring, the sensor should be attached to a finger or earlobe, and it is important to ensure that the measurement site is clean and that blood circulation is not compromised. Every step of the installation requires careful attention, as incorrect application can lead to erroneous readings, compromising patient monitoring and management.

Once the monitoring devices are in place, **continuous monitoring of parameters** becomes an essential task. The caregiver must remain attentive to the data displayed on the monitors, particularly in intensive care units where parameter variations can be rapid and critical. Heart rate, blood pressure, oxygen saturation and respiratory rate are primary indicators that require constant vigilance. In the event of any deviation from normal or expected values, the caregiver must be able to react quickly, alerting the medical team and taking the necessary steps to stabilize the patient. For example, a sudden drop in oxygen saturation may require immediate adjustment of oxygen therapy, while a rapid rise in blood pressure could indicate a hypertensive crisis requiring emergency treatment.

Interpreting monitoring data requires a thorough understanding of normal values and possible variations according to the patient's clinical condition. The caregiver must be able to discern normal physiological changes, such as fluctuations in blood pressure in response to activity or stress, from pathological signs that could indicate a deterioration in the patient's condition. Persistent tachycardia, sudden bradycardia, or irregularities in heart rhythm, for example, need to be assessed in the context of the patient as a whole, not just the numbers on the screen. This ability to interpret data in relation to the patient's clinical condition is what enables the caregiver to play an active role in the healthcare team, contributing to informed decision-making.

In addition to monitoring parameters, **regular checks on the proper functioning of monitoring devices** are essential. The caregiver must ensure that the devices are working properly, that the batteries are sufficiently charged, and that the sensors are not faulty or out of place. Audible and visual alerts from monitors must be taken seriously and checked promptly, as they may indicate a technical problem or medical emergency. Sometimes, interference or artifacts can distort readings, and it's crucial that the caregiver can identify these situations to avoid inappropriate interventions. Cleaning and maintenance of equipment are also part of the caregiver's responsibilities, as clean and well-maintained equipment is essential to ensure accurate and reliable measurements.

Finally, **the communication of monitoring data** is another important dimension of surveillance. The caregiver must clearly and concisely transmit relevant information to nurses and doctors, particularly in the event of significant changes or emergencies. This fluid communication between the different members of the care team enables rapid, coordinated care, essential in an environment where every second can count. In emergency situations, this ability to interpret and communicate monitoring data effectively can mean the difference between life and death.

Post-operative care in cardiology

○ Care after coronary intervention: Angioplasty, bypass surgery, stenting

Care after coronary intervention, whether angioplasty, bypass surgery or stenting, is crucial to ensure optimal recovery and prevent complications. These procedures, although common in cardiology, involve delicate manipulation of the coronary arteries, which are responsible for supplying blood to the heart muscle. After such procedures, rigorous monitoring and careful care are essential to ensure the success of the operation and the stability of the patient.

After a-angioplasty procedure that dilates a blocked coronary artery with a balloon-one of the main concerns is to prevent complications such as restenosis (narrowing of the artery) or stent thrombosis. Monitoring vital signs is essential, including blood pressure, heart rate and oxygen saturation. The caregiver must be particularly vigilant for signs of ischemia, such as chest pain, sudden shortness of breath, or changes in the electrocardiogram (ECG), which could indicate an acute complication requiring rapid intervention. The catheter insertion site, usually in the groin or wrist, should be monitored for signs of bleeding, hematoma or infection. Compression dressings can be applied to minimize the risk of bleeding, and it is important to check the integrity of these dressings regularly.

Stenting, often performed as part of angioplasty, also introduces special considerations. The stent, a small wire mesh tube, is designed to keep the artery open and ensure adequate blood flow. After placement, patients are usually put on antiplatelet therapy to prevent clots from forming in the stent. The caregiver must ensure that the patient takes his or her medication as prescribed, and watch for signs of bleeding complications, which can be a side effect of these treatments. The patient must also be made aware of the importance of adherence to this treatment, as premature discontinuation of antiplatelet drugs can lead to stent thrombosis, a potentially fatal complication.

After coronary **artery bypass grafting (CABG) - a** more invasive surgery that creates a new route to bypass a blocked or narrowed artery - post-operative care is even more intensive. This procedure requires monitoring in an intensive care unit for the first hours to days following the operation. The patient is usually on assisted ventilation until he or she is stable enough to breathe on his or her own. Chest drains, often placed to drain fluid and air from the thoracic cavity, must be carefully monitored to ensure that they are working properly and that drainage is adequate. The caregiver plays a key role in maintaining surgical site hygiene, monitoring for signs of infection, and assessing pain. Effective pain management is essential to enable early mobilization, which is crucial to prevent complications such as pulmonary embolism or pneumonia.

Early mobilization is another important component of care after coronary intervention. As soon as the patient's condition permits, he or she is encouraged to start mobilizing, first by sitting and then by walking. This not only helps prevent thromboembolic complications, but also boosts patient morale and promotes faster recovery. The caregiver should accompany the patient through these first stages of mobilization, ensuring that he or she does not experience excessive pain, dizziness or other alarming symptoms. Progressive, well-supervised mobilization is essential to avoid falls or other incidents.

Patient education is also a crucial aspect of post-operative care. The patient needs to understand the importance of maintaining a healthy lifestyle to avoid further surgery. This includes advice on diet, smoking cessation, stress management and regular exercise. The caregiver plays a key role in conveying this information, ensuring that the patient and family understand the recommendations and are motivated to follow them. The caregiver can also provide practical advice on how to manage care at home, such as administering medication, monitoring for signs of infection, and scheduling follow-up appointments.

Finally, **preparation for discharge and long-term follow-up** are essential to ensure the long-term success of the operation. Before discharge from hospital, the caregiver must ensure that the patient has all the information needed to continue convalescing safely at home. This includes managing medication, monitoring warning signs, and the importance of follow-up consultations. The patient should also be encouraged to participate in a cardiac rehabilitation program, which combines supervised exercise, psychological support, and education on the management of cardiovascular risk factors.

○   Management of thoracic drains

The management of chest drains is an essential post-operative procedure, particularly after heart or lung surgery, such as coronary artery bypass grafting or valve repair surgery. These drains are placed to evacuate fluids, air or blood that may accumulate in the thoracic cavity, thus avoiding potentially serious complications such as pleural effusions, hemorrhage or pneumothorax. The management of these drains requires rigorous attention and specific expertise on the part of healthcare professionals, particularly orderlies, who play a key role in patient follow-up and monitoring.

Installation and initial monitoring of thoracic drains are crucial steps. Once the drain has been inserted by the surgeon, it is connected to a drainage system that operates either by gravity or controlled suction. The caregiver must ensure that the drainage system is correctly configured and that the connections are secure to avoid any risk of accidental disconnection, which could lead to air entering the thoracic cavity and causing a pneumothorax. It is essential to check regularly that the device is working properly, without obstruction, and that the suction level is in line with medical prescriptions.

Continuous monitoring of thoracic drains involves careful control of several parameters. The caregiver must monitor the quantity, color and consistency of the drained fluid, as these provide valuable indications of the patient's condition. For example, a sudden increase in the volume of fluid drained, or a change in its color (such as a more reddish hue indicating possible hemorrhage) should be reported immediately to the medical team. Similarly, a rapid decrease or cessation of drainage may indicate a drain obstruction, requiring rapid intervention to avoid complications.

Dressing management **around the** drain **insertion site** is also a crucial aspect of care. The insertion site must be kept clean and dry to prevent infection. The caregiver should regularly check the dressing for signs of infection, such as redness, swelling or purulent discharge. If a dressing change is necessary, this should be done under strict aseptic conditions to minimize the risk of contamination. In the event of signs of infection, it is crucial to alert the medical team immediately for assessment and appropriate treatment.

Patient mobility is another important factor to manage in the presence of chest drains. While early mobilization is encouraged to prevent complications such as deep vein thrombosis or pneumonia, it is essential to ensure that drains remain secure and functional while the patient is moving. The caregiver should help the patient mobilize safely, ensuring that drainage tubes are not pulled or kinked. Supports or pockets can be used to secure the drains while the patient stands up or walks, allowing some freedom of movement without compromising the function of the drains.

Patient education is also an essential aspect of chest tube management. The patient needs to be informed about the importance of drainage, the signs to look out for, and the precautions to take to avoid any disconnection or obstruction of the system. The caregiver plays a key role in this education, explaining to the patient and family how to manage the drains on a daily basis, particularly if the patient has to return home with the drain still in place. This includes advice on hygiene of the insertion site, how to monitor the drain, and when to contact a healthcare professional in the event of a problem.

Finally, **the removal of the chest tube** is a procedure that also requires special attention. This is usually carried out by a doctor or specialist nurse, but the caregiver often assists with the procedure. Before removal, it is important to ensure that the patient is fully informed of what is going to happen, and that he or she is reassured. After removal, the insertion site must be monitored for any signs of complications, such as air leakage or infection. The dressing should be kept in place and checked regularly to ensure that the site is healing properly.

- Pain management and post-operative complications

Managing post-operative pain and complications is a central component of cardiology patient management, particularly after surgery or an invasive procedure. After an operation such as coronary bypass, stenting or angioplasty, the patient's body is under considerable stress, and careful monitoring is required to ensure that recovery takes place in the best possible conditions. Caregivers play a key role in this process, as they are on the front line in assessing, relieving and preventing complications, while ensuring the patient's comfort.

Managing post-operative pain is one of the first challenges after surgery. Pain can vary depending on the type of operation, but is often significant after major surgeries such as coronary artery bypass grafting. It can affect not only the patient's comfort, but also his or her ability to breathe deeply, mobilize, and actively participate in rehabilitation. For this reason, proactive and effective pain control is essential.

The caregiver contributes to this management by regularly monitoring the intensity of pain felt by the patient, often using pain scales (such as the numerical or visual scale) to assess the level of suffering. Open communication with the patient is essential, as it helps to tailor treatment to the patient's needs. Pain management is often based on a multimodal approach, which includes the administration of prescribed analgesics (oral or intravenous) as well as non-pharmacological techniques such as gentle mobilization, relaxation, or the application of cold or heat to painful areas. The caregiver ensures the correct administration of treatments and that side effects, such as drowsiness or constipation, are also monitored and managed.

Early mobilization of the patient, although sometimes painful at first, is crucial to prevent post-operative complications such as deep vein thrombosis or pneumonia. After cardiac surgery, the chest pain associated with the sternal incision can restrict the patient's movements and deep breathing, increasing the risk of respiratory complications. The caregiver should gently encourage the patient to start moving as soon as his or her condition allows, accompanying him or her on initial movements and ensuring that regular breathing exercises are performed to promote lung expansion.

Respiratory complications are a major concern after surgery, especially in bedridden patients or those who have undergone incisions in the thorax. The risk of pneumonia or atelectasis (partial collapse of the lungs) is high if patients are not mobilized or do not take deep breaths. Caregivers play a key role in preventing these complications by encouraging regular use of the incentive spirometer, a device that helps patients take deep breaths, and reminding them to cough to clear their airways. This helps to keep the lungs open and prevent the build-up of secretions, thereby reducing the risk of infection.

Thromboembolic complications, such as deep vein thrombosis (DVT) or pulmonary embolism, are also frequent risks after surgery, especially in patients confined to bed for long periods. Prevention involves not only early mobilization, but also the use of compression stockings, monitoring for signs of DVT (such as pain, swelling or redness in the legs), and sometimes the introduction of preventive anticoagulation. The caregiver must be vigilant for these signs and ensure that the prescribed preventive measures are put in place, while at the same time making the patient aware of the importance of moving his or her legs regularly while bedridden.

Infectious complications are another important area to monitor, particularly at incision sites or chest drains. The orderly plays a crucial role in infection control by maintaining rigorous hygiene of surgical sites, observing signs of infection (redness, discharge, swelling or fever), and ensuring the cleanliness of dressings. If an infection is suspected, it is essential to alert the medical team immediately so that rapid antibiotic treatment can be initiated or local care adjusted.

Cardiovascular complications, such as arrhythmias, hypotension or hypertension, can occur following the procedure and must be closely monitored. The nursing auxiliary is often responsible for regularly monitoring vital parameters such as blood pressure, heart rate and oxygen saturation. Any significant deviation from normal values should be reported promptly, as it may indicate a potential complication requiring prompt medical intervention.

Finally, **psychological management of** the patient is an essential dimension of post-operative care. Many patients experience anxiety, fear or depression after surgery, particularly as they become aware of the seriousness of their condition and the long-term changes to their lifestyle. The caregiver, through his or her constant presence, can offer emotional support, reassuring the patient, listening to his or her concerns, and encouraging the patient to express his or her emotions. This psychological dimension is just as important as physical care, as it contributes directly to the patient's overall well-being and ability to participate actively in his or her rehabilitation.

Managing cardiological emergencies

○   Recognizing the signs of a heart attack

Recognizing the signs of a heart attack is an essential skill for any healthcare professional, especially in a cardiology department where rapid intervention can save lives. A heart attack, or myocardial infarction, occurs when blood flow to part of the heart muscle is interrupted, usually due to an obstruction in one or more coronary arteries. This prevents oxygen from reaching the heart muscle, leading to irreversible damage if the problem is not treated quickly. For the caregiver, being able to spot the first signs of a heart attack is crucial to alerting the medical team and initiating emergency treatment.

The most common symptom of a heart attack is chest pain. This pain is generally described as a sensation of pressure, squeezing, or heavy weight on the chest, located behind the breastbone. Unlike other types of pain, it does not disappear with rest and can last for several minutes, sometimes more than 20. It can occur suddenly or gradually, and is often felt as an intense, oppressive pain that can radiate to other parts of the body, such as the left arm, neck, jaw or back. This type of pain, known as retrosternal pain, is a major indicator of a heart attack, and it is essential that the caregiver is alert to these descriptions on the part of the patient.

However, **not all patients experience this typical pain.** Symptoms can vary considerably from one person to another, particularly in women, the elderly and diabetics, who may present more atypical symptoms. In these patients, chest pain may be absent or less marked, but other signs may appear, such as **difficulty in breathing** (dyspnea), sudden **intense fatigue**, or a **feeling of general malaise**. These signs are often less recognizable, but they should alert the caregiver, especially if the patient has a history of cardiovascular disease.

Cold sweats, often associated with a heart attack, are another sign to watch out for. These are profuse sweats, sometimes accompanied by clammy, pale skin, which appear suddenly, unrelated to physical activity or ambient temperature. This sweat is often the result of activation of the autonomic nervous system in response to cardiac stress, and may be accompanied by a feeling of anxiety or panic. If a patient complains of excessive sweating, particularly associated with chest pain or shortness of breath, this should be taken very seriously.

Shortness of breath is also a frequent symptom in heart attack patients. The patient may experience difficulty in breathing, even at rest, sometimes with a feeling of suffocation or tightness. This shortness of breath is often due to the heart's inability to pump blood efficiently throughout the body, resulting in a build-up of fluid in the lungs, known as pulmonary edema. Caregivers must be particularly alert to any signs of unexplained dyspnea, as it may precede or accompany a heart attack.

Nausea and vomiting can also be signs of a heart attack, although they are less familiar to the general public. These symptoms are more frequently observed in women, and may be associated with a feeling of indigestion or gastric reflux. It is therefore important not to underestimate them, especially if they are accompanied by other more typical signs, such as chest pain or shortness of breath.

Finally, **palpitations or sensations of irregular heartbeat** may indicate that a heart attack is underway. If a patient reports a sensation of rapid, irregular heartbeat, or describes a sensation of "fluttering" or disordered heartbeat, this may be a sign of an infarct-related arrhythmia. These arrhythmias, such as ventricular fibrillation, can be fatal if not treated immediately. The caregiver must monitor these signs and alert the medical team promptly if a patient complains of such symptoms.

        ◦   Cardiopulmonary resuscitation (CPR) techniques
Cardiopulmonary resuscitation (CPR) is an essential emergency technique that can save lives in the event of cardiac arrest. When

cardiac arrest occurs, the heart stops pumping blood efficiently, depriving the body, particularly the brain, of oxygen. Without rapid intervention, irreversible brain damage can occur within minutes, and death is inevitable without resuscitation. CPR aims to maintain minimal blood circulation and oxygenation until the heart can be restarted by more advanced methods, such as defibrillation. For caregivers, mastering CPR is an indispensable skill, as their speed and efficiency in performing these gestures can make all the difference to a patient's survival.

Basic cardiopulmonary resuscitation (or BLS, Basic Life Support) consists of two main elements: chest compressions and mouth-to-mouth insufflations, although recent recommendations favor chest compressions alone in some cases, particularly for lay rescuers. Chest compressions are the central element of CPR, as they maintain minimal blood flow to vital organs, notably the brain and heart.

Chest compressions should be performed vigorously and evenly. The caregiver, or other rescuer, should kneel beside the victim lying on a flat, hard surface. Once it has been determined that the person is unresponsive and not breathing normally, compressions begin immediately. The hands should be placed one on top of the other, in the center of the chest, just on the midline of the sternum. The rescuer uses the heel of his or her hand to apply firm, continuous pressure to the chest, ensuring that each compression depresses the chest by about 5 to 6 centimeters for an adult. The frequency of compressions is equally important: they should be performed at a rate of 100 to 120 compressions per minute, which corresponds to a fairly fast tempo.

It is essential that compressions are not only deep, but also regular, with a full return of the chest between each compression, to allow the heart to fill with blood before the next compression. The quality of compressions is paramount, as too-light or irregular compressions considerably reduce the chances of successful resuscitation. The caregiver must also ensure that

55

compressions are not interrupted, unless defibrillation is required or the rescue team takes over.

Inflations, or artificial ventilation, are the second component of traditional CPR. They are performed after each cycle of 30 chest compressions. To administer effective insufflations, the paramedic must open the patient's airway by gently tilting the head back and lifting the chin. Next, the rescuer pinches the victim's nose, covers the mouth completely with his or her own, and blows steadily into the victim's lungs for about a second, just long enough for the chest to rise. Two insufflations should be performed after each series of 30 compressions. It's crucial not to blow in too much air or too quickly, as this could cause the stomach to swell and lead to vomiting, complicating resuscitation.

In certain situations, particularly in the event of cardiac arrest on a public road or with an unknown patient, current CPR recommendations for non-professional rescuers favor chest compressions without insufflations (the so-called "hands-only" technique). This method is easier to implement for untrained people, and remains effective in the short term for maintaining minimal circulation until help arrives.

The use of an automated external defibrillator (AED) is also an integral part of modern CPR. When an AED is available, it should be used as soon as possible, as defibrillation is often the only effective way to restart a heart in ventricular fibrillation, one of the main causes of cardiac arrest. The AED is designed to be simple to use, and can be operated by non-medical personnel. The caregiver places the adhesive electrodes on the patient's chest as indicated by the device, which then automatically analyzes the heart rhythm. If a shock is required, the AED issues the instruction to move away from the patient before sending the electric shock. This shock can restore a normal heart rhythm if the arrest is due to ventricular fibrillation or ventricular tachycardia.

During resuscitation, **it is essential to watch for signs of renewed spontaneous cardiac activity**, such as movement, regular breathing or detectable pulses. The caregiver must be ready to adapt his or her intervention as the patient's condition evolves, while ensuring that resuscitation procedures are carried out without major interruption until emergency medical assistance arrives or normal circulation is resumed.

Post-resuscitation management is just as crucial. If the patient regains consciousness or shows signs of life after resuscitation, it is important to continue monitoring vital functions, including breathing and pulse, until the medical team takes over. The patient should be placed in the lateral position to keep the airway clear and prevent the risk of vomiting or choking.

     o Management of acute lung edema

The management of acute pulmonary edema (APE) is a frequent medical emergency in cardiology, requiring rapid and effective intervention to prevent serious, even fatal complications. Acute lung edema is a condition in which fluid rapidly accumulates in the lungs, compromising the alveoli's ability to exchange oxygen. This accumulation of fluid is usually due to acute heart failure, where the heart is unable to pump blood efficiently, causing stasis in the pulmonary circulation. As this pressure increases, fluid seeps into the alveoli, causing severe respiratory distress. Managing this situation requires an immediate response from the care team, with the caregiver playing an essential role in monitoring, supporting the patient, and applying the first therapeutic gestures.

The first clinical signs of acute lung edema are often dramatic, and need to be quickly identified. The patient presents with intense dyspnea, often accompanied by a feeling of suffocation or choking. This difficulty in breathing is often aggravated when lying down (orthopnea), forcing the patient to sit up or sit up straight to try to catch his or her breath. The patient may also exhibit cyanosis (bluish coloration of the lips and extremities) due to reduced oxygenation of the blood, as well as profuse, cold sweating, a sign of the impending state of shock. Auscultation

57

often reveals bilateral crackling rales, especially at the base of the lungs, reflecting the presence of fluid in the pulmonary alveoli. Another characteristic sign is the production of frothy, sometimes pinkish sputum, the result of fluid and blood mixing in the respiratory tract.

When acute lung edema is suspected, **immediate management** is based on a series of rapid actions designed to relieve the patient's respiratory distress and stabilize his or her condition. One of the first interventions is to place the patient in a sitting or semi-seated position (Fowler), which facilitates breathing by reducing pressure on the lungs. The caregiver must reassure the patient, who is often in great distress, while preparing the equipment needed for the treatment.

The administration of high-concentration oxygen is a priority for improving patient oxygenation. A high-concentration mask is generally used to deliver oxygen continuously, with the flow rate adjusted to maintain oxygen saturation above 90%. In the most severe cases, assisted ventilation may be required, notably using non-invasive positive pressure ventilation (CPAP or BiPAP) to reduce the workload on the heart and lungs. This technique improves gas exchange by keeping the airways open and forcing air into the pulmonary alveoli, thus preventing alveolar collapse and fluid re-accumulation.

The administration of diuretics, such as furosemide, is another mainstay of treatment for acute lung edema. Diuretics help eliminate excess fluid by increasing urinary excretion, thus reducing the fluid overload that causes edema. The caregiver must closely monitor the effects of diuretics, paying particular attention to urine output, as a rapid increase in diuresis is a sign of treatment efficacy. It is also crucial to watch for signs of dehydration or an excessive drop in blood pressure, which can occur in response to excessive diuresis.

Blood pressure management is also a central aspect of acute pulmonary edema treatment, especially if the underlying heart failure is due to a hypertensive crisis. In many cases, rapid vasodilation is required to reduce pressure in the pulmonary vessels. Vasodilator drugs such as trinitrin can be administered to dilate blood vessels, thereby reducing the heart's filling pressure and blood stasis in the lungs. The caregiver should carefully monitor the patient's blood pressure to ensure that it remains within acceptable limits, as these drugs can cause a sudden drop in blood pressure.

Continuous monitoring of vital parameters is crucial throughout care. The caregiver should frequently measure respiratory rate, oxygen saturation, blood pressure and heart rate. Any significant change, such as a sudden drop in oxygen saturation or persistent tachycardia, should be reported immediately to the medical team, as this may indicate a worsening of the patient's condition. In addition, it's important to watch for signs of relief, such as improved breathing or reduced patient anxiety, which may indicate that the treatment is working.

If the patient's condition worsens, particularly if there are signs of cardiogenic shock (severe hypotension, cold clammy skin, weak thready pulse), more invasive measures may be required, such as intubation and mechanical ventilation. In these situations, the caregiver must be ready to assist the medical team in setting up resuscitation equipment, and to continue monitoring the patient's immediate needs.

Post-critical management of acute lung edema involves ongoing monitoring once the crisis has stabilized. The patient remains under observation to prevent recurrence, and therapeutic adjustments are often necessary to manage underlying heart failure or other factors that caused the edema. The caregiver continues to play an essential role in monitoring vital parameters, managing diuresis, and educating the patient on how to take their medication and prevent future decompensation.

Chapter 3

Daily care and patient support in cardiology

The caregiver's role in hygiene and comfort care

  ◦   Mobilization techniques for cardiac patients
Mobilization techniques for cardiac patients are an essential part of their post-operative and rehabilitation care. After cardiac surgery, myocardial infarction or cardiac decompensation, gradual recovery of mobility is essential to prevent complications associated with prolonged bed rest, such as deep vein thrombosis, pulmonary infections or muscle wasting. Early mobilization also plays a key role in cardiac rehabilitation by improving blood circulation, promoting better lung function, and helping patients regain their independence. However, mobilization of cardiac patients must be carried out with caution, taking into account their clinical condition and physical capacity, and ensuring that specific protocols are followed to avoid over-exertion or the risk of falling.

Passive mobilization is often the first step for the most fragile patients, especially those who have just undergone major surgery, such as coronary bypass, or who are still in intensive care. In these cases, the patient is not yet able to move independently, and it is the caregiver who gently mobilizes the patient's limbs to prevent joint stiffness and maintain blood circulation. This technique involves gentle, slow movements of the patient's arms and legs, avoiding excessive stress on the thorax, especially if a sternal incision is present. Passive movements limit the risk of complications associated with immobility, while respecting the recovery process. These movements must be performed regularly, taking into account the patient's tolerance, and without causing pain.

As the patient's condition improves, we move on to **assisted active mobilization**, where the caregiver accompanies the patient in his or her first efforts to move. This phase is often initiated shortly after the operation, sometimes as early as the next day, depending on the patient's general condition and medical recommendations. The aim is to encourage the patient to perform light movements, such as lifting an arm or leg, while providing

62

physical support to ensure safety. Assisted active mobilization enables the patient to start using his or her muscles without tiring excessively. During this phase, the caregiver must closely monitor signs of fatigue or shortness of breath and adjust the patient's efforts accordingly.

Bedside mobilization, often referred to as "chair sitting", is a key step in the rehabilitation process. This technique involves helping the patient to sit upright at the edge of the bed, then transferring to a chair. This may seem a simple step, but it is crucial in preparing the patient to stand and walk again. For the cardiac patient, who may still be weak and vulnerable to dizziness or orthostatic hypotension, this transition must be carried out with care. The caregiver should be alert to signs of discomfort, such as dizziness or accelerated heart rate, and offer physical support, often by placing an arm around the patient's back or using a patient lift if necessary. This technique gradually increases tolerance to sitting and prepares the patient for standing.

Once the patient is able to sit up without difficulty, we move on **to active standing mobilization and assisted walking**. This phase is crucial for strengthening the muscles and restoring the patient's autonomy. The caregiver then helps the patient to stand up, ensuring that his or her legs can bear the weight of the body without wobbling. The patient may be helped by the use of a cane, a walker, or simply the caregiver's arm to provide support and maintain balance. Walking is gentle, over short distances, often around the bed or in the hallway, with frequent breaks to avoid fatigue. The caregiver must be particularly attentive to signs of cardiac fatigue, such as shortness of breath, chest pain or palpitations. If such signs appear, it's important to stop walking immediately and allow the patient to rest.

Gradual adaptation of effort is a key principle in the mobilization of cardiac patients. It is important never to push the patient beyond his or her limits, as excessive effort can trigger symptoms of heart failure or angina (chest pain). Each stage of mobilization must be evaluated according to the patient's response. The caregiver must be able to assess the clinical condition in relation to vital parameters (such as heart rate, oxygen saturation and blood pressure), and know how to adapt the pace of exercise or movement to keep the patient in a zone of comfort and safety.

Alongside these physical mobilizations, it is also essential to encourage the patient to perform **breathing exercises**, often with the help of an incentive spirometer. These exercises help to improve lung function, increase respiratory capacity and prevent lung infections. The caregiver must guide the patient through these exercises, ensuring that they are performed correctly and regularly, especially after cardiac surgery.

The psychological aspect of mobilization must also be taken into account. Many heart patients, especially those who have just undergone major surgery or suffered a heart attack, may be reluctant to move, for fear of tiring themselves out or worsening their condition. The caregiver's role here is to accompany and motivate, reassuring patients and gradually encouraging them to regain confidence in their physical abilities. A caring and encouraging attitude is essential to encourage mobilization, which can be perceived as a challenge for anxious or depressed patients after their operation.

○ Hygiene care for patients with medical devices (catheters, probes, etc.)

Hygiene care for patients with medical devices, such as catheters, probes or drains, is essential to ensure their comfort, prevent infections and guarantee the proper functioning of the devices. These patients require special attention, as the presence of these devices increases the risk of complications, particularly nosocomial infections. Caregivers play a key role in managing daily hygiene, while taking care to respect the specific features of each medical device. Appropriate hygiene care helps maintain good personal hygiene, while ensuring that devices are protected and maintained.

The first fundamental principle of hygiene care for patients with medical devices is asepsis: catheters, probes and other invasive devices create potential entry points for infectious agents. As a result, every treatment must be carried out under rigorous conditions of cleanliness. Before any care, the caregiver must wash his or her hands thoroughly with hydroalcoholic solution or antiseptic soap, and in many cases, wear non-sterile gloves. It is essential to handle devices with care, avoiding contact with contaminated surfaces and minimizing unnecessary handling of devices.

Patients with central venous catheters (CVCs) or peripheral venous **catheters**, for example, require adapted hygiene care that takes into account the need to protect the catheter insertion site. During daily cleansing, it is important to avoid wetting the dressing covering the insertion site. If the patient is able to shower, a waterproof protective film can be applied to protect the catheter area. The caregiver should check the dressing regularly to ensure that it is clean, dry and securely in place. If the dressing becomes soiled or detached, it must be changed under aseptic conditions to avoid contamination. Monitoring the insertion site for signs of infection, such as redness, pain or discharge, is also a priority.

For patients with **urinary catheters**, perineal hygiene is particularly important to prevent urinary tract infections, a frequent complication associated with these devices. The caregiver must perform careful intimate hygiene, using lukewarm water and mild soap, gently cleaning the area around the catheter outlet, without pulling on the device. This cleansing should be carried out at least once a day, and whenever necessary (after incontinence, for example). It is also crucial to check that the urinary drainage system remains below the level of the bladder to avoid any reflux, and that the tubing is not kinked or obstructed, to ensure proper urine flow.

Patients with **surgical drains**, placed to drain fluids after surgery, require special hygiene care around the drain exit site. The caregiver must ensure that the skin around the drain is clean and free from irritation or signs of infection. As with catheters, it is important not to wet the drain area while washing. The caregiver must also monitor the drainage system, ensuring that fluid is draining properly and reporting any changes in the color, quantity or odor of the drained fluid, which could indicate a complication.

Hygiene care for patients with **nasogastric tubes** or gastrostomies (for enteral feeding) also requires particular vigilance. The skin around the tube orifice must be kept clean and dry to avoid irritation or infection. The caregiver should gently clean the skin around the tube with lukewarm water and mild soap, taking care not to move or pull the tube. For nasogastric tubes, it is also important to monitor the patient's nose and throat for signs of irritation or infection, and to ensure that the tube attachment remains in place to avoid any accidental displacement or discomfort.

Patients with **implanted pacemakers or automatic defibrillators** also require appropriate hygiene care, particularly in the days or weeks following the procedure. The incision should be protected when washing, and the caregiver should check that the area is clean and that there are no signs of infection or device rejection, such as redness, pain or swelling around the implanted area.

Finally, another important aspect of hygiene care for patients with medical devices **is patient education**. The caregiver plays a crucial role in explaining to the patient how to maintain personal hygiene while caring for their device. This includes practical advice on grooming, the importance of reporting any pain or changes around the device, and what to avoid doing to prevent complications (such as accidentally pulling or moving the device). This education enables patients to actively participate in their own care, and reduces the risk of infection or device malfunction.

◦   Pressure sore prevention in bedridden patients

Preventing pressure sores in bedridden patients is a top priority in nursing care, particularly in cardiology, where many patients may be immobilized after a procedure or due to their fragile state of health. Pressure sores, also known as pressure ulcers, are skin lesions caused by prolonged pressure on an area of the body, usually at support points such as the heels, sacrum or hips. This pressure prevents proper blood circulation, depriving tissues of oxygen and nutrients, which can lead to cell death and wound formation. An untreated pressure sore can develop into a serious infection, even septicemia, and compromise the patient's recovery. Pressure sore prevention is based on a series of measures designed to reduce pressure, protect the skin and encourage mobilization, as far as the patient's condition allows.

The first step in preventing pressure sores is regular mobilization of the patient. Bedridden patients, especially those in intensive care or following surgery, need to be mobilized as frequently as possible to prevent pressure from building up on pressure points. When the patient's mobility is limited, it is essential to reposition him or her every two hours to change the distribution of pressure on the body. The caregiver must take care to lift the patient gently, using sliding sheets or support cushions, to avoid pulling or rubbing the skin, which could aggravate the risk of injury. Mobilization is not just about changing position in bed; encouraging the patient to sit at the edge of the bed, to get up, or to use a chair, depending on their state of health, also helps to reduce the risk of pressure sores.

The use of pressure-relieving devices is another key strategy for preventing pressure sores. Special mattresses and cushions, such as dynamic air mattresses or viscoelastic foam cushions, are designed to distribute pressure evenly over the whole body and relieve pressure points. These devices help reduce the pressure exerted on vulnerable areas, allowing better blood circulation in the tissues. The caregiver must ensure that these devices fit and function correctly, while regularly checking their effectiveness against the patient's condition. For patients at high risk of pressure

67

sores, particularly those who are very thin or have poor circulation, the use of heel supports to relieve pressure on the feet and ankles is particularly recommended.

Regular assessment of the patient's **skin** is essential to detect the first signs of pressure sores and take immediate action. Caregivers should inspect at-risk areas such as the sacrum, heels, hips, elbows and shoulder blades daily, looking for redness, areas of heat or hardened skin, which are early warning signs of a pressure sore. Persistent redness that does not blanch under pressure is a warning sign that a skin lesion is forming. If these signs are detected, it's crucial to intervene quickly by relieving pressure on the affected area and reinforcing preventive measures, such as using extra cushions or repositioning more frequently.

Skin care also plays a central role in pressure sore prevention. Well-moisturized, clean skin is less vulnerable to lesions. Caregivers must ensure that bedridden patients maintain rigorous hygiene, with daily cleansing and particular attention to areas at risk of maceration, such as skin folds or areas around medical devices. The use of gentle, hypoallergenic and moisturizing products is essential to avoid any irritation or excessive dryness of the skin, which could encourage the formation of bedsores. In addition, for incontinent patients, it's crucial to change pads frequently and clean the skin after each incontinence episode, to prevent maceration and irritation, which greatly increase the risk of pressure sores.

Nutrition also plays a fundamental role in pressure sore prevention. A balanced diet, rich in proteins, vitamins and minerals, is essential to maintain skin health and promote healing. Patients confined to bed or recovering from heart surgery may be at risk of malnutrition, which weakens the skin and makes it more vulnerable to damage. The caregiver must ensure that the patient receives a diet adapted to his or her needs, in collaboration with the dietician, and monitor any signs of malnutrition or weight loss. If necessary, nutritional supplements may be recommended to support healing and strengthen skin resistance.

Patient and family education is another important aspect of pressure sore prevention. The caregiver can explain to the patient and family the importance of mobilization, skin care and nutrition in preventing pressure sores. For patients who will be bedridden at home, it is crucial to provide practical advice on repositioning techniques, the use of specialized cushions or mattresses, and regular skin monitoring. By actively involving patients and their families in preventive care, we reinforce their autonomy and reduce long-term risks.

Psychosocial support for patients and their families

- The importance of active listening and empathetic communication

The importance of active listening and empathic communication in healthcare, particularly in cardiology, cannot be overstated. These interpersonal skills play a fundamental role in the quality of care, patient support and the creation of an environment of trust and well-being. In a medical context where patients may feel anxious, fearful or uncertain about their state of health, active listening and empathic communication not only meet their emotional needs, but also improve understanding and adherence to treatment. By being close to patients on a day-to-day basis, the caregiver is often the first person to whom patients turn to express their concerns, doubts or suffering. The way in which these exchanges are managed can have a considerable impact on the patient's quality of life and care pathway.

Active listening is much more than simply hearing what the patient is saying. It involves total attention, concentration on the words and emotions being expressed, and an ability to perceive what is not being said directly, such as signs of distress, discomfort or frustration. When caregivers practice active listening, they show the patient that they are fully present and engaged in the exchange. This is demonstrated by simple but meaningful gestures, such as looking the patient in the eye, nodding slightly, and asking open-ended questions that encourage the patient to think more deeply. By adopting this attitude, the caregiver sends a clear message: "What you feel and what you have to say is important to me". This strengthens the relationship of trust, encouraging the patient to feel understood and respected.

Empathic communication, on the other hand, is based on the ability to put oneself in the patient's shoes and understand his or her experience, without judgment. It involves recognizing the patient's emotions, whether explicit or underlying, and responding appropriately. In cardiology, where patients may experience moments of great vulnerability - for example, after a diagnosis of heart disease, an operation or a critical episode such as a heart attack - empathy is essential to offer them moral support. Empathic communication creates a space in which patients feel free to express their fears, pain or frustrations, in the knowledge that their emotions will be received with kindness. The caregiver can express this empathy in simple but powerful phrases, such as: "I understand how difficult this must be for you", or "It's normal to feel worried after what you've just been through". These words, though simple, bring immense comfort to the patient, who then feels cared for as a whole, and not just on a medical level.

Active listening and empathetic communication also improve therapeutic adherence. When patients feel listened to and understood, they are more likely to follow medical recommendations and become actively involved in their own treatment. For example, a patient who feels supported and encouraged by the healthcare team will be more likely to comply with post-operative instructions, participate in cardiac rehabilitation sessions, or take their medication regularly. On the other hand, a patient who feels ignored or misunderstood may develop a distrust of the nursing staff, or even a sense of disengagement from his or her own treatment, which can compromise recovery.

Managing difficult emotions is another area where active listening and empathic communication play a crucial role. Cardiology patients, often faced with the seriousness of their condition, can be overwhelmed by intense emotions, such as fear of death, anxiety about an uncertain future, or anger at the loss of autonomy. By listening actively and showing empathy, the caregiver can help defuse, channel and calm these emotions. The aim is not to minimize the patient's suffering, but to offer them a space where they feel safe to express their feelings. It also helps to establish a constructive dialogue on the emotional aspects of treatment, which sometimes tend to be neglected in favor of purely medical considerations.

Active listening and empathic communication also promote better collaboration within the care team. When caregivers take the time to listen and offer empathic support, they are able to gather valuable information about the patient's emotional and psychological state, which they can then pass on to other members of the medical team. This fluid, empathic communication improves care coordination and enables treatment to be tailored more comprehensively, taking into account both the physical and emotional needs of the patient. The caregiver thus becomes an essential link between the patient and the care team, ensuring that the patient's needs are fully taken into account.

◦   Managing stress and anxiety in patients

Managing stress and anxiety in patients is an essential component of medical care, particularly in cardiology, where patients may be faced with situations of great uncertainty, pain or fear. Stress and anxiety can have a significant impact on patients' physical and mental health, and are often exacerbated by the diagnosis of serious illnesses, such as cardiac pathology, or by the prospect of surgery. For the caregiver, understanding and managing these emotions is crucial not only to improving the patient's emotional well-being, but also to promoting a better response to treatment and a faster recovery.

The causes of stress and anxiety in patients are varied and often multifactorial. They may be linked to uncertainty about diagnosis, fear of medical intervention, physical pain, or fear of the long-term consequences of illness. In cardiology, for example, a patient who has just suffered a myocardial infarction may experience profound anxiety linked to the possibility of a recurrence or the loss of physical capacity. The perception of a loss of control over one's body and health often aggravates this feeling of anxiety. What's more, hospitalization itself, with its unfamiliar surroundings, noises and disrupted rhythms, can accentuate stress, especially for patients who feel isolated from their families and daily lives.

One of the first steps in managing stress and anxiety in patients is to establish a climate of trust through open, empathetic communication. The caregiver must be available and attentive to the patient's concerns, giving them the opportunity to express their fears and worries freely. Active listening plays an essential role here: it enables the caregiver to gather not only the patient's complaints and questions, but also the underlying emotions, such as anxiety or frustration. By responding empathetically and without judgment, the caregiver helps the patient to feel heard and understood, which often reduces the intensity of anxiety. For example, reassuring a patient about the progress of a procedure, or clearly explaining the next steps in treatment, can alleviate some of their worries and give them back a sense of control.

Relaxation techniques are also highly effective in helping patients manage stress. The caregiver can introduce simple deep breathing or progressive muscle relaxation exercises, which help the patient to reduce nervous tension and regain a sense of inner calm. Deep breathing, in particular, helps to regulate heart rate and improve oxygenation, which is particularly beneficial for cardiac patients. By guiding the patient through these techniques, the caregiver offers a concrete tool that the patient can use when feeling a surge of stress or anxiety, whether in hospital or after discharge.

The care environment plays an important role in managing stress and anxiety. A calm, clean and organized environment can help to calm patients. The caregiver can help create this environment by limiting unnecessary noise, adjusting lighting to make it less aggressive, and ensuring that the patient has all the elements necessary for comfort (cushions, blankets, etc.). Allowing the patient access to familiar objects, such as photos, or means of distraction (reading, music) can also help reduce feelings of isolation and stress.

Managing pain-related stress is another essential dimension in the management of anxious patients. Pain is often a major source of anxiety, especially when the patient anticipates future pain or has already suffered intense pain. The caregiver must be attentive to the patient's complaints and ensure proactive pain management by administering prescribed treatments, monitoring their efficacy and adjusting care according to the patient's needs. Poorly controlled pain can not only aggravate anxiety, but also delay recovery, as it encourages the patient to avoid mobilization or resist certain treatments. By providing effective pain relief, the caregiver helps to reduce stress and improve the patient's quality of life during hospitalization.

Involving family and friends in managing the patient's stress is also beneficial. Social support plays a crucial role in the emotional well-being of hospitalized patients. The caregiver can facilitate contact with the family, organize visits or suggest means of communication (telephone, videoconferencing) to maintain the link with loved ones. These interactions reassure patients and help them to cope better with hospitalization. What's more, involving the family in explanations of care or medical decisions reinforces the feeling of security and support.

In some cases, it may be necessary to involve professionals specializing in stress and anxiety management. If the patient presents significant anxiety that interferes with his or her ability to cooperate with care or to recover, the caregiver can refer to a psychologist or psychiatrist, who can suggest appropriate therapeutic approaches, such as cognitive-behavioral therapy or the prescription of anxiolytics. These interventions are particularly useful for patients suffering from chronic anxiety or post-traumatic stress disorders.

Finally, **patient education** is a key dimension in anxiety management. The more a patient understands about their illness, treatment and recovery, the less stress they will feel. The caregiver can play an important role by explaining medical procedures in simple, understandable language, providing information about medication and reassuring the patient about the positive effects of treatment. This education empowers the patient and gives them a sense of control over their situation, which significantly reduces anxiety.

◦　　Support for families in critical situations
Supporting families in critical situations is an essential aspect of hospital care, particularly in departments such as cardiology, where patients can experience moments of great vulnerability. Whether it's a heart attack, major surgery or an unforeseen complication, families often find themselves destabilized, faced with anxiety, uncertainty and the fear of losing a loved one. In these critical moments, the role of the caregiver and the nursing team is not limited to caring for the patient; it also includes providing human and empathetic support for families, who are also affected by the seriousness of the situation. Appropriate support can not only alleviate their emotional suffering, but also strengthen their resilience and enable them to accompany the patient more serenely through the care process.

Welcoming families in crisis situations is a crucial first step. As soon as an emergency or complication is announced, the caregiver must ensure that families are received in a calm, secure environment. It's important to create a space where they feel listened to and supported. In a stressful situation, families need clear information and friendly human contact. The caregiver, as a privileged intermediary, can take the time to explain the situation, avoiding drowning loved ones in incomprehensible technical details, but giving them a reassuring overview. A simple gesture, such as offering a chair, a glass of water, or a quiet place to rest, can help calm the first few minutes of an anxious situation.

Communication is at the heart of family support. At critical moments, uncertainty is often what fuels the anxiety of loved ones. They want to understand what's going on, how the patient's condition is evolving, and what the next steps are. The caregiver must ensure that families receive regular information, even if the situation is still being assessed. Honest, clear and empathetic communication is essential. Families need to know that they can ask questions at any time, and that no question is trivial. Sometimes it's helpful to rephrase medical information to make sure everything has been understood and to avoid misunderstandings. Empathy must permeate every interaction: even in a difficult situation, the caregiver can reassure families that everything is being done to care for the patient.

Emotional support is another key component of family support. When a patient's condition is critical, emotions can run high: fear, anger, sadness, sometimes feelings of helplessness. The caregiver must be able to recognize these emotions and respond with compassion. Active listening plays an essential role here. Allowing families to express their feelings, doubts or even anger without judgment is a way of supporting them in their emotional process. In some cases, it can be helpful to encourage them to talk about their concerns, to externalize their stress, and to verbalize how they feel. This dialogue, though sometimes emotionally charged, can be a valuable outlet for loved ones. The caregiver can also suggest the presence of a psychologist or spiritual advisor for those who feel the need for more in-depth support.

Involving families in medical decisions is another important aspect of support in critical situations. If the patient is critically ill and unable to express themselves, families are often involved in difficult decisions about care. The caregiver, although not directly responsible for medical decisions, can play a vital role in explaining options, answering questions, and helping to clarify aspects of treatment. This involvement is essential if families are not to feel excluded or powerless in the face of the situation. Giving them a role, however modest, in the decision-making process reinforces their sense of usefulness and involvement, which can alleviate their stress.

Supporting families in the face of uncertainty is a delicate but necessary task. During critical periods, there may be prolonged periods of waiting when little information is available, particularly when a patient is in the operating theatre or intensive care unit. These waiting periods are often the most trying for loved ones. The caregiver can alleviate this anxiety by assuring them that they will be informed immediately of any changes in the patient's condition, offering them regular follow-up, even if there is no new information to share. This helps families to feel cared for and not left in total uncertainty.

Managing the most critical moments, such as the announcement of a reserved prognosis or death, requires special attention. In these situations, the caregiver, alongside the doctor, must accompany the family with profound humanity. The announcement of tragic news must be made with delicacy, leaving time for loved ones to understand and assimilate what has just happened. It is crucial to offer a space of intimacy and respect, and to allow families to deal with their grief in their own way. The caregiver can also help by answering the practical questions that often arise at these moments, such as organizing visits or managing the administrative aspects of the medical aftermath.

Finally, **post-crisis support** is just as important. Once the critical situation has passed, whether resolved or not, families still need support. If the patient recovers, they will need to be guided through the next stages of rehabilitation, understand the care to be provided, and prepare for an eventual return home. If the outcome is more tragic, the caregiver needs to ensure that families are put in touch with support services, such as a palliative care service, psychologist or support groups. This post-crisis follow-up is essential to ensure that loved ones are not left alone to face their grief or the challenges that arise after a critical period.

Nutrition in cardiology

      °   Dietary principles for cardiac patients

Dietary principles for cardiac patients play a fundamental role in the prevention, management and recovery from cardiovascular disease. An appropriate diet not only helps to improve heart health, but also reduces the risk of complications and recurrence, and promotes a better quality of life. Patients suffering from heart disease, such as hypertension or heart failure, or after a heart attack, need to adopt specific dietary habits to control risk factors such as cholesterol, blood pressure and body weight. Caregivers, in conjunction with dieticians and doctors, have an important role to play in educating and supporting patients so that they can implement these dietary principles in their daily lives.

One of the basic principles of diet for heart patients is to reduce consumption of saturated and trans fats. These types of fat, found mainly in animal products (fatty meats, cold meats, butter, cream) and processed foods (fried or ultra-processed industrial products), are directly linked to increased levels of LDL cholesterol, also known as "bad cholesterol". An excess of this type of cholesterol promotes atherosclerosis, a build-up of plaque in the arteries, which can lead to heart attack or stroke. For heart patients, it is therefore recommended to favor unsaturated fats, found in vegetable oils (olive, rapeseed), avocados, walnuts and oily fish (such as salmon or mackerel), which have protective effects on cardiovascular health. Omega-3s, in particular, present in these foods, have anti-inflammatory properties and help regulate heart rhythm.

77

Reducing salt (sodium) intake is another fundamental principle for heart patients, especially those with high blood pressure. Excessive salt consumption contributes to water retention in the body, which increases blood volume and, consequently, the pressure exerted on artery walls. This can worsen hypertension and force the heart to work harder, ultimately leading to heart failure. General recommendations for heart patients are to limit sodium intake to around 1,500 mg a day, equivalent to one teaspoon of salt. This restriction means paying attention to processed foods, often rich in hidden salt, such as ready-made meals, industrial sauces, and even certain breads and cereals. To enhance the flavour of dishes without using salt, we recommend using aromatic herbs, spices or citrus fruits, which add flavour without harming heart health.

Increasing dietary fiber intake, particularly soluble fiber, is also essential as part of a cardioprotective diet. Soluble fibers, found in fruits, vegetables, legumes (such as lentils, beans or chickpeas), and whole grains (oats, barley), help reduce blood cholesterol levels by binding to bile acids in the intestine, thus promoting their elimination. This reduces cholesterol absorption and helps prevent the build-up of plaque in the arteries. What's more, fiber helps regulate blood sugar levels, which is particularly important for heart patients who also suffer from diabetes, as optimal blood sugar control is crucial in preventing cardiovascular complications.

Portion control and calorie management are also important, especially for overweight and obese patients. Being overweight is a major risk factor for cardiovascular disease, as it increases the heart's workload and favours the development of hypertension, diabetes and high cholesterol. Adopting a balanced diet, but also watching portion sizes, helps to lose weight or maintain a healthy weight, which in turn helps to take the strain off the heart. Heart patients should be encouraged to adopt regular meals, well distributed throughout the day, while avoiding caloric excess, particularly from fast sugars, which promote weight gain and glycemic imbalances.

Hydration is another crucial aspect of dietary principles for heart patients. Adequate hydration helps maintain good blood volume and support cardiac function. However, in heart failure patients, it is often necessary to monitor fluid intake to avoid fluid overload, which could worsen their condition. In such cases, fluid restriction may be recommended, and it is essential that patients follow their medical team's advice on how much water to consume on a daily basis. Caregivers must also ensure that patients understand the importance of limiting beverages high in sugar, caffeine or sodium, such as sodas or energy drinks, which can be deleterious to heart health.

Antioxidants, vitamins and minerals, found in a diet rich in fresh fruit and vegetables, also play a protective role. These foods, rich in vitamins (such as vitamin C and E), potassium, magnesium and flavonoids, contribute to cardiovascular health by reducing inflammation, improving endothelial function and regulating blood pressure. Potassium, in particular, helps counterbalance the effects of sodium on blood pressure. It is therefore recommended that heart patients consume a wide variety of fruit and vegetables every day, ideally at least five portions, to reap their nutritional benefits.

Finally, **patient education and support in implementing these dietary principles are essential**. For many patients, changing their eating habits can be difficult, especially if their food culture or family habits are deeply rooted. The caregiver, in collaboration with the dietician, plays a key role in educating and supporting patients, helping them to understand the importance of these dietary adjustments and offering practical solutions for adapting their diet. This can include advice on meal preparation, reading food labels, and managing temptations or harmful eating habits. By reinforcing this education, patients can better integrate these changes into their daily lives and improve their long-term health.

◦ Monitoring water intake and fluid balance

Monitoring fluid intake and fluid balance is an essential component of patient care, particularly in cardiology and on wards where patients present with pathologies associated with fluid retention, heart failure, or electrolyte imbalances. Fluid balance, which represents the balance between fluids ingested and those eliminated, is crucial to ensuring proper organ function, maintaining cardiovascular stability, and preventing serious complications such as pulmonary edema, hypertension, or renal failure. The caregiver plays a key role in monitoring this balance, keeping a close eye on fluid intake and output, and ensuring that any imbalances are quickly detected and reported to the medical team.

Fluid intake includes both oral and intravenous fluids, and in patients with heart or renal failure, fluid intake often needs to be strictly controlled to avoid fluid overload, which could worsen their condition. Patients with heart failure, for example, have a reduced capacity to eliminate excess fluids, leading to an increased risk of edema, pulmonary congestion and worsening heart failure. The caregiver must therefore ensure compliance with the instructions given by the medical team regarding the amount of fluids the patient is allowed to drink each day. This may include limiting drinks to a certain amount, as well as monitoring liquids hidden in food (such as soups, water-rich fruits, or jellies).

Fluid balance monitoring is based on tracking fluid inputs and outputs. Inflows include all beverages and fluids administered by infusion, as well as fluids contained in food. Outputs include urine, stools (in the case of diarrhea), vomit, as well as insensible losses (such as perspiration or respiration). To maintain rigorous monitoring, it is important that the caregiver accurately records each intake and output in a monitoring chart or care record. Every liter of fluid consumed or eliminated must be recorded, as even small variations can have major consequences on the patient's condition, especially in those with fragile fluid balance.

Management of fluid output mainly involves urine measurement, which is a key indicator of renal function and fluid balance. In bedridden patients or those with urinary problems, a urinary catheter may be required to accurately measure diuresis (the volume of urine produced over a given period). The caregiver must regularly check the quantity of urine eliminated and ensure that it is in line with the targets set by the medical team. Low diuresis)oliguria) or absence of urine (anuria) may indicate renal dysfunction or fluid retention, and should be reported immediately. Similarly, excessive diuresis (polyuria) may indicate an imbalance, for example linked to the use of diuretics, and requires assessment to adjust treatment.

Signs of fluid overload should also be carefully monitored. Excessive fluid accumulation in the body can lead to edema, particularly in the ankles, feet and sometimes the abdomen. These edemas are often visible as swellings, and pressure exerted on the skin can leave an imprint (cup edema). Caregivers should be alert to these signs, and raise the alarm immediately if such symptoms appear, as they may indicate that the patient is accumulating more fluid than he or she is eliminating. In addition to peripheral oedema, fluid overload can cause breathing difficulties, due to pulmonary oedema, resulting in shortness of breath or crackling rales on auscultation. Rapid weight gain is also a sign of fluid retention. A sudden increase in weight, even modest (e.g. 1-2 kg in a few days), can be an early indicator of overload, and daily weighing of at-risk patients is an effective way of detecting such changes.

Conversely, dehydration can occur if water intake is insufficient or losses are excessive. Dehydration can be particularly dangerous in cardiac patients, as it can reduce blood volume, thereby increasing heart rate and the heart's workload. Clinical signs of dehydration include intense thirst, dry mucous membranes, reduced urine production, orthostatic hypotension (lower blood pressure when standing), and sometimes confusion. The caregiver must monitor these signs and ensure that patients receive adequate hydration according to their individual needs.

Electrolyte balance is closely linked to water balance, particularly for sodium and potassium, which play a key role in regulating heart and kidney functions. Too much or too little fluid can upset the balance of these electrolytes, leading to serious complications. For example, hypokalemia (low potassium) can lead to dangerous cardiac arrhythmias, while hypernatremia (excess sodium) can aggravate dehydration. Caregivers must therefore pay close attention to the results of laboratory tests, especially in patients receiving diuretics or undergoing strict fluid restriction.

Educating patients and their families about managing fluid intake is an essential aspect of long-term follow-up, particularly after hospitalization. For patients with heart or kidney failure, monitoring fluid intake often has to be continued at home. The caregiver can play a key role in teaching patients how to monitor their own fluid intake and diuresis, how to recognize signs of overload or dehydration, and how to adjust their intake according to medical recommendations. This includes practical advice on how to measure fluids, distribute intake throughout the day, and choose foods that do not promote excessive water retention.

   ○   Collaboration with the dietician for adapted food plans

Collaboration between the nursing auxiliary and the dietician is essential to develop dietary plans tailored to the specific needs of patients, especially those suffering from chronic diseases such as heart disease, diabetes or renal failure. This synergy ensures that nutritional aspects are fully integrated into the care process, with a common goal: to promote recovery, improve quality of life and prevent complications. Each patient has unique dietary needs, and the combined role of the caregiver and dietician is to ensure that these needs are met in an individualized and effective manner.

The dietician's role in this collaboration is to design dietary plans adapted to the patient's specific medical conditions. For example, for a patient suffering from heart failure, the dietician will draw up a plan to limit salt intake to prevent water retention and reduce pressure on the heart. Similarly, for a diabetic patient, a plan will be devised to control carbohydrate intake and avoid major fluctuations in blood sugar levels. The dietician takes into account several factors, such as the patient's age, weight, gender, level of physical activity, food preferences and medical history. Through this detailed analysis, he or she proposes a personalized diet that contributes to improving the patient's overall health, while respecting his or her tastes and habits.

Nurses, for their part, play a key role in implementing and monitoring these dietary plans. They are in direct daily contact with patients, ensuring that dietary recommendations are followed. He helps patients understand nutritional advice, choose the right foods and respect dietary restrictions, especially when patients are hospitalized or have difficulty managing their diet alone. For example, if a patient has strict limitations in terms of sodium or fluid intake, the caregiver ensures that these instructions are respected on a daily basis.

Accompanying patients who are frail or reluctant to change their eating habits is another dimension of the collaboration between caregivers and dieticians. Many patients can feel at a loss when faced with major dietary changes, particularly when these involve foods they have been eating for a long time. The role of the caregiver is to motivate and encourage these patients to gradually integrate these changes into their daily lives, while remaining attentive to their needs and preferences. Working with the dietician, he or she can suggest dietary alternatives that respect both medical requirements and the patient's tastes, making the food plan more appealing and easier to follow.

Ongoing monitoring of the patient's progress is another fundamental aspect of this collaboration. In addition to checking adherence to the diet plan, the caregiver is responsible for monitoring the effects of the diet on the patient's health. This may include monitoring weight, watching for signs of fluid retention or dehydration, or observing any symptoms linked to poor dietary management, such as fluctuations in blood sugar levels in a diabetic patient. When problems are identified, the caregiver can alert the dietician, so that the latter can adjust the diet plan accordingly. For example, if a patient gains or loses weight unexpectedly, or shows signs of nutritional deficiencies, the dietician can reassess the situation and modify the diet according to the patient's needs.

Hospital meals are another area where collaboration between the caregiver and dietician is particularly important. When a patient is hospitalized, meals are often prepared according to specific dietary recommendations. The caregiver must ensure that the meals served correspond to the dietician's recommendations. If the patient has difficulty eating certain foods, or if he or she expresses dietary preferences, the caregiver informs the dietician, who can then adjust the menus accordingly. This communication ensures that the patient does not eat inappropriate foods, or eat too little, which could jeopardize recovery.

Long-term patient education is an essential component of this collaboration. The aim of dietary management is not only to meet the patient's immediate needs during hospitalization, but also to help them adopt sustainable eating habits that will promote their long-term health. The caregiver, with the support of the dietician, plays a key role in educating patients about the basic principles of their diet. This includes practical advice on how to prepare meals at home, read food labels, plan balanced meals, and deal with situations where food temptations or family habits might interfere with their diet.

Finally, **raising awareness among the** patient's **family and friends** is also part of this collaborative approach. Relatives often play an important role in managing patients' diets, especially after they have returned home. The caregiver and dietician can organize information sessions for families, to make them aware of the patient's nutritional needs and give them tips to help them follow their meal plan. This helps to create a family environment conducive to compliance with dietary instructions, which is essential to avoid relapses or complications.

Chapter 4

Prevention and Therapeutic Education in Cardiology

The caregiver's role in preventing complications

  ◦   Prevention of nosocomial infections in cardiology
Preventing nosocomial infections in cardiology is an absolute priority to ensure patient safety and quality of care. Nosocomial infections, also known as healthcare-associated infections, occur in healthcare establishments and are contracted by patients during hospitalization. They can have serious consequences, especially in cardiology, where patients are often fragile due to underlying medical conditions such as heart failure, a history of infarction, or following surgery such as coronary bypass or stenting. Preventing these infections relies on a series of strict measures, from hand hygiene to the rigorous management of medical devices such as catheters, probes and drains. The involvement of the entire health-care team, including orderlies, is essential to limit risks and protect patients.

Hand hygiene is one of the simplest and most effective measures for preventing nosocomial infections. In cardiology, where many patients are immunocompromised or vulnerable to infection, systematic and rigorous hand washing is essential. Hands can easily transmit germs, especially when in contact with contaminated surfaces or after caring for another patient. It is therefore essential that caregivers and all healthcare staff wash their hands before and after any contact with a patient, before performing an invasive procedure (such as catheter insertion), and after touching potentially contaminated surfaces. The use of hydroalcoholic solutions is particularly recommended, as they are fast, effective and well tolerated by the skin. Caregivers should also make patients and their families aware of the importance of hand hygiene, by offering them hydroalcoholic solutions to use before touching the patient or his or her immediate environment.

The management of invasive medical devices is another key aspect of infection prevention in cardiology. Patients hospitalized in cardiology may have devices such as central or peripheral venous catheters, urinary catheters or chest drains. These devices, although necessary, are potential entry points for infections. Every manipulation must therefore be carried out under strict aseptic conditions. For example, when caring for a catheter, it is crucial to disinfect the insertion site thoroughly and to change dressings regularly. The caregiver plays a key role in monitoring insertion sites, checking for redness, heat, discharge or other signs of infection, and reporting any abnormalities immediately. Urinary catheters, for example, must be handled with clean gloves, avoiding contamination of the drainage system.

Sterilization of medical equipment is another essential preventive measure. All equipment used in cardiology, whether surgical tools, catheters or probes, must be sterile to prevent the transmission of germs. Caregivers must ensure that all equipment is clean and properly sterilized before use, and that reusable instruments are decontaminated after each use. Strict compliance with sterilization and disinfection protocols is essential to prevent infections associated with the use of contaminated equipment.

Hygiene of premises and surfaces is also crucial to prevent the spread of germs in the patient's environment. In the hospital environment, many surfaces (bedside tables, carts, door handles, etc.) can be contaminated by pathogens. The caregiver must therefore ensure the cleanliness of the patient's environment by making sure that surfaces are cleaned and disinfected regularly, especially in high-risk areas such as intensive care units. Monitoring devices, beds and shared medical equipment must be cleaned after each use. In addition to regular cleaning, it is essential to ensure that patient rooms are ventilated and maintained in hygienic conditions to limit germ proliferation.

Antibiotic stewardship is also a key component in the fight against nosocomial infections, in particular to avoid the selection of antibiotic-resistant bacteria. In cardiology, patients may receive prophylactic antibiotics, for example before surgery, to prevent infection. However, excessive or inappropriate use of antibiotics can encourage the development of resistant strains, making infections more difficult to treat. It is therefore essential to comply with medical prescriptions and rigorously monitor antibiotic treatments to ensure they are administered under the right conditions. The nursing auxiliary must also ensure that patients scrupulously follow their treatment and that antibiotics are not prematurely discontinued without medical advice.

Training and awareness-raising for healthcare staff are fundamental aspects of preventing nosocomial infections. Care practices are constantly evolving, and it is essential that all staff, including orderlies, are regularly trained in new procedures and infection prevention protocols. This includes training in the correct use of personal protective equipment (PPE) such as gloves, masks, gowns and safety glasses, which are essential in certain situations to protect both patients and staff. In addition, regular workshops on good hygiene practices serve as a reminder of the importance of each daily gesture in the fight against infections.

Surveillance and management of epidemics in cardiology departments are also part of preventive measures. In the event of a confirmed or suspected nosocomial infection, it is essential to quickly isolate the patient concerned to avoid spreading the infection to other patients, particularly those already compromised by their cardiac condition. Caregivers must be trained to identify the early signs of nosocomial infections, whether surgical wound infections, nosocomial pneumonia or urinary tract infections, and to implement isolation measures when necessary. Prompt, rigorous management of infections helps to limit their spread and ensure the safety of all patients.

○ Monitoring thromboembolic complications

Monitoring for thromboembolic complications is a crucial part of care, particularly in cardiology, where many patients are at increased risk of blood clots. These complications, such as deep vein thrombosis (DVT) or pulmonary embolism (PE), can have serious or even fatal consequences if not detected and treated promptly. Blood clots can occur in bedridden patients, after surgery, or in the presence of heart conditions such as atrial fibrillation, which increase the risk of abnormal blood flow and stasis. For the caregiver, monitoring for early signs of thromboembolic complications is essential to prevent these events and ensure prompt, effective management.

Deep vein thrombosis (DVT) is one of the most common thromboembolic complications, particularly in patients who are hospitalized or immobile for long periods. It generally occurs in the deep veins of the lower limbs, where a blood clot can form due to venous stasis, vascular trauma or hypercoagulability. Caregivers must be alert to the early signs of DVT, as it can rapidly progress to pulmonary embolism if the clot migrates to the lungs. Classic signs of DVT include swelling, pain or tenderness in the calf or thigh, a sensation of local heat, and sometimes redness or hardening of the skin over the affected area. Unilaterality of these symptoms (affecting only one limb) is a key clue, and any sudden change in the appearance or sensation of the limb should be reported immediately. Monitoring these signs is particularly important in bedridden patients, after surgery or post-partum, where the risk of DVT is increased.

Pulmonary embolism (PE) is the most serious complication of DVT, as the clot formed in a deep vein can break loose and travel to the lungs, blocking blood flow and compromising oxygenation. Untreated pulmonary embolism can lead to cardiorespiratory arrest. Clinical signs of pulmonary embolism include sudden dyspnea (difficulty in breathing), acute chest pain which may worsen on deep inspiration, tachycardia, cyanosis (bluish discoloration of the lips and extremities), and coughing, sometimes accompanied by hemoptysis (coughing up blood). Caregivers must be particularly attentive to these symptoms, especially if the patient has a history of DVT or risk factors such as prolonged immobilization. Any sudden deterioration in respiratory status or unexplained chest pain should be regarded as potential emergencies, requiring immediate alerting of the medical team.

The prevention of thromboembolic complications relies heavily on early mobilization and the use of compression devices. For bedridden patients, one of the most effective measures for preventing clot formation is regular mobilization. Caregivers should encourage patients to move as soon as their condition allows, by helping them to stand up and walk, or, if this is not possible, by performing passive mobilization exercises of the lower limbs. Simple exercises such as plantar and dorsal flexion (flexion and extension of the ankles) help maintain active blood circulation in the legs. For patients unable to mobilize, the use of intermittent pneumatic compression devices or compression stockings is another essential measure. The caregiver must ensure that these devices are correctly used, adjusted and tolerated by the patient, and regularly check that they remain in place and functional.

Monitoring anticoagulant therapy, frequently used to prevent thromboembolic complications, is also a key aspect of care. At-risk patients, especially those with arrhythmias such as atrial fibrillation or who have undergone surgery, are often given anticoagulants to prevent clots from forming. Caregivers must ensure that these drugs are administered as prescribed, and monitor any side effects, such as bleeding. Anticoagulants increase the risk of bleeding, and the appearance of unexplained bruising, bleeding gums, traces of blood in the urine or stools, or vomiting with blood are warning signs. Monitoring for signs of bleeding is therefore essential to balance the protective effect of anticoagulants against the risk of bleeding.

Monitoring clinical and biological parameters is also an important part of preventing and monitoring thromboembolic complications. The caregiver can contribute to this monitoring by regularly checking the patient's vital parameters, such as heart rate, blood pressure and oxygen saturation, especially in patients at risk of pulmonary embolism. A sudden drop in oxygen saturation, unexplained tachycardia or a fall in blood pressure should alert you to a possible complication. In addition, biological tests such as the INR (International Normalized Ratio), which measures the effectiveness of blood coagulation under anticoagulant treatment, must be closely monitored. If the INR is too high, the risk of bleeding increases, while an INR that is too low may signal ineffective treatment, leaving the patient vulnerable to thrombosis.

Patient education is an important aspect of preventing thromboembolic complications. Patients need to understand the measures they can take to reduce their risk, including regular mobilization, wearing compression stockings if prescribed, and taking their anticoagulant medication as directed. The caregiver plays an essential role in this education, explaining to the patient the importance of these measures and answering any questions they may have. For example, for patients coming out of surgery or with a history of DVT, it's crucial to explain why it's important to keep moving, even after they've been discharged from hospital, and to comply with medical prescriptions, even if symptoms have subsided.

In conclusion, monitoring for thromboembolic complications is a task of prime importance in the hospital environment, particularly for bedridden, post-operative patients or those with cardiovascular risk factors. By being attentive to the first clinical signs, ensuring that preventive measures are correctly applied and monitoring anticoagulant treatments, the nursing auxiliary contributes directly to the prevention of these serious complications. Through their hands-on role and involvement in the day to-day care of patients, they play an essential role in the early detection and effective management of thromboembolic complications.

○   Relapse prevention and long-term monitoring
Relapse prevention and long-term monitoring are essential pillars in the management of cardiology patients, particularly after serious events such as myocardial infarction, cardiac surgery or an episode of decompensated heart failure. Once patients have passed through the acute phase of their treatment, the aim is to

prevent any further deterioration in their state of health. This prevention is based on a healthy lifestyle, compliance with medication and regular medical supervision. The caregiver, as a front-line player in patient follow-up, plays a crucial role in this long-term prevention, supporting the patient on a daily basis and helping him/her to maintain health habits that reduce the risk of relapse.

Lifestyle modification is one of the fundamental aspects of relapse prevention. After a cardiac episode or surgery, patients often need to review their daily habits to better manage risk factors. This includes stopping smoking, reducing alcohol consumption, adopting a suitable diet, and integrating regular physical activity. The caregiver, in conjunction with other healthcare professionals, can encourage and support the patient in making these changes. The aim is not only to provide practical advice, but also to reinforce the patient's motivation to adopt these new habits, which are sometimes difficult to maintain. For example, a patient who is having difficulty giving up smoking may benefit from psychological support or the guidance of a tobaccologist. Similarly, the caregiver can work with the dietician to adapt the patient's diet, taking into account his or her preferences, to ease the transition to a healthier diet.

Compliance with medication is another pillar of relapse prevention. Most heart patients require long-term medication, whether to control blood pressure, regulate cholesterol or prevent blood clots. The caregiver can play a key role in ensuring that the patient takes his or her medication correctly, in the prescribed doses and at the prescribed times. In some cases, patients may be reluctant to take their medication, either because they don't fully understand its importance, or because of the side effects. The caregiver can then clearly explain why each drug is necessary to prevent a relapse, and alert the doctor to any difficulties or poor tolerance. This vigilance is crucial, as non-adherence to medication can rapidly lead to a destabilization of the patient's state of health.

Adapted physical activity is also a key element in relapse prevention. After a heart attack or heart surgery, cardiac rehabilitation, which includes a supervised exercise program, is often recommended. These exercises improve the patient's physical condition, strengthen the heart and reduce the risk of recurrence. The caregiver, in collaboration with physiotherapists and doctors, can encourage the patient to take an active part in these programs. Once the rehabilitation program has been completed, it is crucial that the patient continues to maintain a regular level of physical activity, adapted to his or her abilities. The caregiver can provide advice on appropriate types of exercise, such as walking, cycling or swimming, and encourage the patient to incorporate these activities into his or her daily routine.

Stress management and psychological support are also key factors in relapse prevention. Many cardiac patients suffer from anxiety or depression after an acute episode, which can hinder their recovery and increase the risk of future complications. By listening and being present on a regular basis, the caregiver can help the patient express his or her concerns and find strategies to better manage stress. They can also refer patients to specialized resources, such as support groups or psychologists, if necessary. In addition, certain relaxation techniques, such as deep breathing or meditation, can be taught to patients to help them stay calm and reduce their stress levels on a daily basis.

Long-term medical monitoring is essential to prevent relapses and detect any signs of destabilization at an early stage. Regular consultations with the doctor or cardiologist enable risk factors to be monitored, treatments to be adjusted if necessary, and the patient's overall state of health to be reviewed. As an intermediary between the patient and the medical team, the caregiver can facilitate this monitoring by observing clinical signs and encouraging the patient to keep medical appointments. They are also responsible for monitoring certain health parameters on a daily basis, such as blood pressure, weight or heart rate, and reporting any abnormalities. For example, sudden weight gain may be a sign of fluid retention in a patient with heart failure, while an irregular heartbeat may indicate uncontrolled atrial fibrillation. In these situations, prompt intervention can prevent a worsening of the patient's condition.

Ongoing patient and family education is also part of long-term prevention. It is essential that patients and their families understand the issues associated with their condition, and are able to recognize the warning signs of a potential relapse, such as chest pain, sudden dyspnea, or excessive fatigue. The caregiver can contribute to this education by clearly explaining the symptoms to watch out for, and giving advice on how to react in an emergency. This helps the patient and family to feel more confident, and to act quickly if necessary.

Finally, **creating a supportive environment** is a key factor in successful relapse prevention. Family and social support play a crucial role in maintaining healthy lifestyle habits and adherence to treatment. The caregiver can help involve the family in care, encouraging them to support the patient in his or her efforts to adopt a healthier lifestyle. A patient surrounded by loved ones who understand his or her needs and encourage him or her to stay active, eat healthily and adhere to treatment is more likely to succeed in preventing a relapse.

Educating patients about their disease and treatment

> ○ Explanation of drug treatments: beta-blockers, anticoagulants, diuretics, etc.

Explaining drug treatments is a crucial step in patient management, particularly in cardiology, where drugs play a key role in managing cardiovascular disease, preventing complications and improving quality of life. Cardiac patients are often faced with a combination of drug treatments that they must follow over the long term, and it is essential that they understand not only the importance of each drug, but also how it works, its side effects and the precautions to be taken. Caregivers, in collaboration with doctors and pharmacists, are involved in this education to ensure that patients comply with their treatment and are able to manage their therapy on a daily basis. Here's an explanation of the main types of medication commonly used in cardiology: beta-blockers, anticoagulants and diuretics.

Beta-blockers are one of the most frequently prescribed classes of drugs in cardiology. They are used to reduce the heart's workload by lowering heart rate, heart muscle contraction force and blood pressure. By blocking the action of stress hormones such as adrenalin on the heart's beta receptors, these drugs help control hypertension, prevent angina pectoris (chest pain linked to insufficient blood supply to the heart), and reduce the risk of recurrence after a myocardial infarction. They are also used to treat certain cardiac arrhythmias, such as atrial fibrillation, where the heart beats irregularly and rapidly. By slowing the heart rate, beta-blockers enable the heart to beat more calmly and efficiently.

Beta-blockers are often well tolerated, but they can cause side effects such as excessive fatigue, dizziness and sometimes bradycardia (an excessive slowing of the heart rate). It's important for patients to understand that they should never abruptly stop this treatment, as this could cause a "rebound", i.e. a sudden increase in heart rate and blood pressure, which can be dangerous. The caregiver must explain to patients that these drugs are essential for long-term heart protection, and that it is necessary to adhere to the prescribed doses.

Anticoagulants, on the other hand, are drugs that prevent the formation of blood clots. They are particularly important in patients at increased risk of thrombosis, such as those with atrial fibrillation, those who have undergone heart surgery, or patients with an artificial heart valve. Clots can lead to serious complications, such as stroke or pulmonary embolism. By thinning the blood, anticoagulants reduce the risk of these clots forming and causing blockages in arteries or veins.

There are several types of anticoagulant, including direct oral anticoagulants (such as rivaroxaban or apixaban), and K-vitamins (such as warfarin). Antivitamins K require stricter follow-up, with regular blood tests to monitor the INR (International Normalized Ratio), which measures treatment efficacy. Anticoagulants carry an increased risk of bleeding, and it's crucial that patients are made aware of this potential complication. The caregiver should explain how to recognize signs of bleeding, such as abnormal bruising, blood in the urine, frequent nosebleeds or black stools. In the event of these symptoms, it is essential to consult a doctor without delay. The caregiver must also stress the importance of never abruptly stopping this treatment without medical advice, even if the patient is feeling well.

Diuretics, often referred to as "water pills", are used to eliminate excess fluid in the body, helping to reduce pressure on the heart. They are commonly prescribed to patients suffering from hypertension, heart failure or edema (fluid build-up in the legs or lungs). By increasing urine production, diuretics help reduce blood volume, thereby lowering blood pressure and easing the strain on the heart to pump blood. There are different types of diuretics, such as loop diuretics (furosemide), thiazide diuretics (hydrochlorothiazide) and potassium-sparing diuretics (spironolactone).

One of the most common side effects of diuretics is the loss of potassium, a mineral essential for heart function. Patients therefore often need to monitor their potassium intake and, in some cases, take supplements if necessary. The caregiver should explain to the patient how to recognize signs of electrolyte imbalance, such as muscle cramps, fatigue or palpitations, and the importance of reporting these symptoms to the doctor. It is also important to explain to patients that, even if they need to urinate more frequently, they should not limit their fluid intake without medical advice, as this could worsen their state of dehydration and lead to complications. Diuretics can also cause dizziness or falls due to the drop in blood pressure, particularly when changing position, which the caregiver must monitor closely, especially in elderly patients.

Other drugs commonly used in cardiology include angiotensin-converting enzyme (ACE) inhibitors, such as ramipril, and angiotensin II receptor blockers (ARBs), such as losartan. These drugs work by relaxing blood vessels, thereby lowering blood pressure and reducing the heart's workload. They are often prescribed after a myocardial infarction or in cases of hypertension. The caregiver must watch out for potential side effects, such as a dry cough (often associated with ACE inhibitors) or dizziness linked to lower blood pressure. It is also important to explain to the patient that these drugs must not be stopped without consulting a doctor, as this could lead to a dangerous rise in blood pressure.

○ Encourage compliance and explain side effects
Encouraging compliance and explaining side effects are two essential aspects of patient management, particularly in cardiology. Therapeutic compliance, i.e. a patient's ability to take medication as prescribed, is a key factor in improving clinical outcomes, preventing complications and promoting a better quality of life. However, it is often difficult for patients to maintain optimal compliance over the long term, not least because of the complexity of treatments, side effects, or a lack of understanding of the real benefits of treatment. The role of the caregiver is fundamental in accompanying, encouraging and sensitizing patients to the importance of their treatment, while providing clear and accessible information on side effects and how to manage them.

The importance of therapeutic compliance lies in the fact that drug treatments, particularly in cardiology, are designed not only to relieve immediate symptoms, but also to prevent serious complications, such as heart attacks, strokes or heart failure. Yet many patients interrupt or modify their treatment without medical advice, either because they don't feel an immediate improvement,

97

or because of troublesome side effects. The caregiver, by virtue of his or her proximity to the patient, is well placed to explain that the effectiveness of treatments, particularly in chronic illnesses, is often seen over the long term. For example, a patient suffering from hypertension may not feel the direct benefits of an anti-hypertensive medication, but it is essential to make them understand that this treatment protects their heart and arteries by reducing the risk of future complications.

To encourage patient compliance, **it is crucial to make the patient the actor in his or her own treatment**, by clearly explaining the objectives of the treatment and establishing an open dialogue about his or her concerns. The caregiver can act as an intermediary between the patient and the medical team, gathering information on obstacles to compliance. For example, some patients may find it difficult to understand how and when to take their medication, especially when faced with complex prescriptions involving several drugs at different times of the day. In this case, the caregiver can help them organize a simplified plan for taking their medication, such as using a pillbox or adopting fixed routines for each dose, to make treatment easier to follow.

Active listening is also a crucial skill in encouraging patient compliance. Patients often express doubts or concerns about their treatment, especially if it has troublesome side effects. The caregiver must listen to these concerns and offer appropriate explanations. For example, a patient on beta-blockers who experiences fatigue or a slowing heart rate may be tempted to reduce the dose or stop treatment. In this case, it's important to explain that these side effects are common at the start of treatment, but often diminish over time. It's also important to remember that beta-blockers help protect the heart by reducing its workload, and that abruptly stopping the medication could lead to a resurgence of symptoms, or even an increased risk of heart attack.

Explaining side effects is another key dimension of the therapeutic relationship, as it helps patients to anticipate and manage these effects, rather than suffer them in silence. It's important for the patient to know that most drugs, although effective, can have undesirable effects, but that these should not discourage him or her from continuing treatment. The caregiver can explain, for example, that certain anticoagulants, such as warfarin, increase the risk of bleeding, and that it is therefore necessary to watch for signs of unusual bruising or bleeding gums. On the other hand, they should be reassured that, under medical supervision, these effects are manageable, and that they should not interrupt their treatment without consulting a professional.

The management of side effects must also be approached proactively. Sometimes, dose adjustments or a change of medication may be necessary to improve treatment tolerance. The caregiver can encourage the patient to report any troublesome side effects, even if they seem minor, as this may indicate that the treatment needs to be reassessed by the doctor. On the other hand, some side effects can be mitigated by simple measures. For example, a patient on diuretics who suffers from muscle cramps due to potassium loss may benefit from dietary advice (such as increasing potassium-rich foods) or the prescription of supplements. By informing the patient about possible solutions, the caregiver helps to improve adherence to treatment and reinforce the patient's confidence in his or her care team.

Therapeutic education plays a central role in improving compliance. For patients to follow their treatment rigorously, they need to understand not only how to take their medication, but also why they are taking it. The caregiver can make medical information accessible by using concrete examples that speak to the patient. For example, by explaining to a hypertensive patient that his antihypertensive medication reduces the pressure on his arteries to prevent them from hardening and clogging, the caregiver transforms an abstract prescription into a concrete gesture to prevent heart attacks or strokes. This approach reinforces understanding and adherence to treatment.

Finally, **involving family and friends** can be a decisive factor in encouraging patient compliance. Relatives often play a moral and logistical support role, helping patients to organize their medication intake or encouraging them to keep up with medical appointments. The caregiver can involve them in discussions about treatment, ensuring that they understand what is at stake and the potential side effects. By creating a supportive environment around the patient, we increase their chances of following their treatment correctly over the long term.

o   Techniques for autonomous symptom management at home

Autonomous symptom management at home is an essential component for patients with chronic diseases, particularly in cardiology. After hospitalization or the acute phase of their illness, patients are often faced with the need to monitor their own health on a daily basis. This can include managing symptoms such as breathlessness, fatigue, chest pain or fluctuating blood pressure. To succeed in this self-management, it is crucial that patients are well informed, equipped and supported to respond appropriately to their body's warning signals and prevent complications. The caregiver plays a fundamental role in educating and preparing patients so that, when they return home, they can monitor their health with confidence and efficiency.

Home therapeutic education is the first step in enabling patients to manage their symptoms independently. It is essential that patients understand what signs to look out for, how to interpret them, and what actions to take in response to each situation. The caregiver, in collaboration with the doctor and other healthcare professionals, can explain the main symptoms that should alert the patient. For example, in a patient suffering from heart failure, signs such as rapid weight gain, increased shortness of breath or swelling of the legs may indicate fluid retention, a sign of cardiac decompensation. The caregiver must inform the patient that these symptoms require a rapid response, either by consulting a doctor immediately, or by adjusting certain aspects of the patient's treatment, as previously agreed with the medical team.

Self-monitoring of vital parameters is one of the most important techniques for autonomous symptom management at home. It involves encouraging patients to regularly measure key health indicators, such as blood pressure, heart rate, weight and oxygen saturation. For cardiac patients, monitoring blood pressure and weight is particularly important. Rapid weight gain over a few days can be an early sign of fluid retention, requiring a reassessment of treatment. Similarly, blood pressure that is too high or too low may signal a need for medication adjustment. The caregiver can train the patient in the use of measuring devices, such as blood pressure monitors or scales, and ensure that he or she knows how to interpret the results properly. It is also important to keep a health diary in which the patient records his or her daily measurements and symptoms, in order to monitor the evolution of his or her condition and provide this information to his or her doctor at follow-up consultations.

Home medication management is another key dimension of autonomous symptom management. Patients undergoing chronic treatment, including cardiac therapies such as beta-blockers, anticoagulants or diuretics, need to follow a strict medication routine to prevent any worsening of their condition. The caregiver can help the patient organize his or her medication by using pillboxes or automated reminders (via mobile apps or alarms), to ensure that he or she doesn't miss any doses. In addition, it's crucial to explain to patients the importance of adhering to dosage and not adjusting their medication on their own, even if they're feeling better or experiencing side effects. In case of doubt, patients should be encouraged to consult their doctor before making any changes.

Recognizing and managing early symptoms is another key aspect of autonomy. In addition to monitoring vital parameters, patients must learn to listen to their bodies and identify the first signs of possible decompensation. The caregiver can explain to the patient how to recognize symptoms that require an immediate response. For example, persistent chest pain or pain radiating to the left arm, accompanied by sweating and nausea, may be the sign of a myocardial infarction, requiring emergency treatment. Similarly, increased shortness of breath or difficulty in breathing while lying down may be a sign of worsening heart failure. Patients should be aware of the steps to take in the event of serious symptoms: contact emergency services immediately or call their GP, depending on the severity of the situation.

Managing lifestyle at home is also crucial to preventing recurrences and stabilizing the patient's condition. The caregiver must encourage the patient to adopt a suitable diet, maintain a moderate level of physical activity and manage stress. For example, when it comes to diet, it's essential that the patient knows the basics of a heart-healthy diet: limit salt intake to avoid fluid retention, favor unsaturated fats such as olive oil, and include more fruit, vegetables and whole grains. The caregiver can provide practical advice on how to integrate these eating habits into the patient's daily routine, and suggest strategies for dealing with temptations or social constraints.

Physical activity, adapted to the patient's state of health, is also beneficial for improving blood circulation and strengthening the heart. The caregiver can recommend simple activities such as walking, cycling or swimming, while explaining the importance of respecting the limits imposed by the patient's state of health. It's important that the patient knows how to adjust his or her effort according to his or her capabilities, and is able to identify signs of over-exertion, such as excessive fatigue or palpitations, and react accordingly by reducing the intensity of exercise.

Emotional and psychological support is an integral part of independent symptom management. Many patients, especially those with chronic illnesses such as heart failure or after a heart attack, may experience anxiety or depression. These emotions can affect their ability to manage their illness effectively and stay motivated to follow their treatment. By listening to the patient's concerns, the caregiver can encourage them to express their feelings and seek psychological support if necessary. They can also refer patients to support groups or specialist services where they can talk to others in similar situations. Good psychological support helps patients to come to terms with their illness and remain proactive in managing their symptoms.

Finally, **communication with the medical team** is essential for successful independent symptom management at home. Patients need to know when and how to contact their doctor or another member of their care team if they have any doubts or worrying symptoms. The caregiver can help the patient prepare questions to ask during follow-up consultations, and organize regular monitoring to adjust treatments as the condition evolves. This ongoing communication helps to avoid complications and to maintain personalized, tailored care.

Cardiac rehabilitation support

       ◦   Encourage the resumption of adapted physical activity

Encouraging the resumption of appropriate physical activity is a fundamental aspect of rehabilitation for cardiac patients and those suffering from chronic diseases. Physical exercise, when properly dosed and adapted to the patient's medical condition, helps to improve cardiovascular health, strengthen muscles and enhance quality of life. After a cardiac event such as a heart attack, surgery or heart failure, physical activity must be resumed gradually, under the supervision of the medical team, in order to prevent complications while providing the expected benefits. Caregivers play an essential role in this process, by raising patients' awareness of the importance of physical activity, motivating them to regain confidence in their abilities, and providing them with the tools to integrate exercise safely into their daily lives.

The importance of physical activity in cardiac rehabilitation is well established. Exercise helps to improve blood circulation, reduce blood pressure, control weight and regulate cholesterol levels. In addition, it promotes better management of stress and anxiety, which are often exacerbated after a cardiac event. One of the key messages the caregiver needs to convey is that even light exercise is an integral part of long-term treatment. Patients need to understand that, in addition to medication and diet, the gradual resumption of appropriate physical activity is a prerequisite for preserving heart health and avoiding recurrences.

Encouraging patients **to resume suitable physical activity** begins with an assessment of their abilities. Depending on the patient's state of health, age, medical history and level of fitness prior to the cardiac event, the activity should be adapted to avoid over-exertion. The cardiac rehabilitation program, often prescribed by the cardiologist and supervised by physiotherapists, is a good starting point. This program is designed to help patients gradually resume exercise, while monitoring their physiological responses, such as heart rate and blood pressure. The caregiver can encourage the patient to take an active part in these sessions, perceiving them as a means of reinforcing their autonomy and increasing their confidence in their physical abilities.

Walking is often one of the first physical activities recommended after a cardiac episode. It's accessible, not too strenuous, and can be adapted to suit all abilities. The caregiver can encourage the patient to walk daily, starting with short distances and gradually increasing duration and intensity as tolerated. Walking not only strengthens heart function, it also improves endurance and blood circulation. To make this activity more enjoyable and motivating, the caregiver can suggest tips such as walking with a loved one, choosing pleasant environments (parks, seaside), or setting progressive targets, for example by using a pedometer to track the number of steps taken each day.

Light muscle strengthening can also be encouraged, especially in patients who have been bedridden for long periods. Prolonged immobility leads to loss of muscle mass and reduced strength, which can make it difficult to resume daily activities. Simple exercises, such as squats, arm lifts or resistance exercises with elastic bands, can help to gradually restore muscle strength. The caregiver can show the patient how to perform these exercises safely, taking care to avoid sudden or overly intense movements, and reminding him or her to breathe properly during the effort.

Adjusting expectations and managing fears are two essential aspects of encouraging the resumption of physical activity. After a cardiac event, patients are often afraid to exercise again, for fear of provoking a recurrence or worsening their condition. The caregiver should reassure the patient that adapted physical activity is not only safe, but also beneficial for the heart, provided it is carried out within the framework of medical recommendations. It can be useful to explain that the body has a great capacity for recovery and that, even if progress is slow, every little effort contributes to strengthening health. The caregiver should also encourage the patient to respect his or her own pace, insisting on the importance of listening to the body and stopping the effort in the event of signs of discomfort, such as chest pain, severe shortness of breath or dizziness.

Variety of activities is another way of making the return to physical exercise more attractive and motivating. Caregivers can suggest a variety of activities to suit the patient's tastes and abilities, such as cycling, gentle swimming, yoga or tai chi. In addition to their physical aspect, these activities often have a relaxing, soothing dimension that can help reduce stress and improve the patient's general well-being. Trying out new activities can also restore the patient's taste for effort, and help them to reintegrate exercise into their daily routine.

Monitoring the body's response to exercise is crucial to ensuring patient safety. The caregiver can encourage the patient to monitor certain parameters during exercise, such as heart rate or fatigue level. For example, the use of a heart rate monitor may be recommended to ensure that the patient does not exceed the heart rate limit set by his or her doctor. It is also important to remind the patient that progress should be gradual, and that any increase in exercise intensity should be discussed with his or her doctor. In the event of worrying symptoms, such as chest pain, severe shortness of breath or dizziness, it is essential to stop the activity and consult a health professional.

Setting realistic, progressive goals is an effective way of maintaining motivation over the long term. The caregiver can help the patient to set personalized goals, such as walking 10 minutes more each week, or reaching a specific number of daily steps. These goals should be adapted to the patient's abilities, and adjusted as progress is made. Establishing regular follow-up with the caregiver or medical team helps to reward the patient's efforts and encourage him or her to persevere.

Finally, **integrating physical exercise into the daily routine** is one of the best ways of ensuring the sustainability of this recovery. It's often easier for patients to maintain regular activity when it's part of their routine. The caregiver can suggest ways of integrating exercise into daily life, such as walking more often instead of taking the car, taking the stairs instead of the elevator, or stretching in the morning. The aim is to make physical activity a natural part of the patient's life, without it becoming a constraint.

- Monitoring and advice during rehabilitation sessions

Monitoring and counseling during rehabilitation sessions are essential elements in helping patients regain full independence after a cardiac event or surgery. Cardiac rehabilitation, in particular, plays a key role in physical recovery, improving cardiac function and preventing recurrence. These sessions, supervised by a multidisciplinary team including cardiologists, physiotherapists and care assistants, enable patients to relearn how to move, strengthen their heart and muscles, while becoming aware of the limits imposed by their state of health. The caregiver, by virtue of his or her proximity to the patient, plays an essential role in this rehabilitation phase: he or she continuously monitors the patient's clinical condition, guides the exercises and, above all, reassures and motivates the patient, enabling him or her to progress in complete safety.

Monitoring vital signs during rehabilitation sessions is crucial to ensure patient safety. Every patient has a different capacity for effort, depending on his or her state of health, and it is essential to constantly monitor certain parameters such as heart rate, blood pressure and oxygen saturation. The caregiver, in conjunction with the physiotherapist, must ensure that these values remain within the limits set by the doctor. For example, after a heart attack or heart surgery, a heart rate that is too high during exercise may indicate that the heart is overloaded. The caregiver can then adjust the intensity of exercise, or ask the patient to take a break to allow the heart to recover. Monitoring vital signs is not just about measuring equipment: the caregiver must also be alert to visible clinical signs such as skin color, shortness of breath, excessive sweating, or the appearance of chest pain.

Adapting exercises to the patient's abilities is another fundamental aspect of rehabilitation sessions. Each patient progresses at his or her own pace, and it is important to adapt the exercises to the patient's level of effort tolerance. For a patient still very weak after surgery or a heart attack, the first sessions may be limited to simple movements, such as slow walking on a treadmill or breathing exercises. The caregiver must be attentive to the patient's reaction to the effort and ensure that it does not exceed his or her capabilities. For example, if a patient feels very tired or dizzy, it is imperative to slow down or stop the exercise to avoid any risk of discomfort. Gradually, as the patient regains strength, exercises can be intensified, with deeper stretching, muscle-strengthening exercises or longer walking times. The caregiver must always bear in mind that rehabilitation is a gradual process, which must be carried out with respect for each patient's abilities and limitations.

Encouragement and managing apprehension play a central role in successful rehabilitation. After a cardiac event, many patients feel anxious about resuming physical activity, for fear of triggering a new cardiac problem. The caregiver must not only monitor the clinical aspects of rehabilitation, but also reassure the patient that physical activity is beneficial to recovery and is supervised to ensure safety. It's important to listen to the patient's fears and answer their questions sympathetically. By explaining that the exercises are specifically designed to gradually strengthen the heart without overloading it, the caregiver helps the patient regain confidence in his or her body. Regular reassurance of the patient, using simple, positive words, plays a fundamental role in allaying fears and maintaining motivation.

Advice on the safe practice of physical activity is essential, not only during inpatient rehabilitation sessions, but also for the continuation of exercise at home. The caregiver can remind the patient of certain important rules, such as the importance of warming up before each exercise to prepare the heart and muscles, or of staying well hydrated before, during and after exercise. It's also important to explain to patients that they should never push themselves beyond their limits, and that they should always listen to their bodies. For example, in the event of chest pain, difficulty breathing or dizziness during exercise, the patient should immediately stop the activity and consult a health professional. The caregiver can also advise the patient on the importance of resting sufficiently between sessions, to give the body time to recover.

Assisting patients to become autonomous is a key objective of rehabilitation sessions. The aim is to help patients feel able to manage their physical activity independently once the supervised sessions are over. The caregiver can suggest simple exercises that the patient can safely do at home, such as daily walking or gentle stretching. They can also explain how patients can monitor their own vital parameters at home, such as heart rate, and record their progress in a logbook. This enables patients to take charge of their own health, while having clear guidelines on what they can do and how far they can go.

Motivation and moral support from the caregiver are also key factors in the success of rehabilitation sessions. It's important to recognize the patient's progress, however modest, and show them that they're moving in the right direction. Regular, positive encouragement builds confidence and keeps the patient engaged in the rehabilitation process. The caregiver may, for example, congratulate a patient for walking longer than the previous week, or for mastering a new exercise. This kind of recognition is essential to avoid discouragement, especially when recovery is long and fraught with difficulties.

Finally, **post-rehabilitation follow-up** is an integral part of long-term monitoring. Once the patient has completed his or her supervised rehabilitation program, he or she must continue to engage in regular physical activity to maintain progress and prevent relapse. The caregiver can provide advice on the type of activities to focus on and how to incorporate them into the patient's daily routine. They can also stress the importance of follow-up consultations with the doctor or cardiologist to adjust the exercise program as the patient's state of health evolves.

- ○ Preparing for the return home and post-hospitalization advice

Preparing patients for their return home and providing post-hospital counseling are crucial steps in their care after a period of hospitalization, particularly in cardiology or after major surgery. A successful transition from hospital to home requires careful planning to ensure that the patient is ready to manage their condition, follow their treatment and continue their recovery in a more independent environment. The caregiver's role in this phase is fundamental, helping to inform, reassure and support the patient and family, ensuring that they have the knowledge and resources they need to avoid complications and optimize recovery.

Psychological and emotional preparation is one of the first steps in preparing for the return home. After hospitalization, especially for a heart condition or surgery, patients may feel anxious about leaving the constant supervision of nursing staff. They may fear they won't be able to manage their treatment on their own, or recognize the signs of a complication. The caregiver plays an important role in allaying these fears. He or she must explain to the patient that returning home is a positive sign of their recovery, and that care will continue at home, with resources available should the need arise. Good emotional preparation also means ensuring that the patient knows who to turn to in case of doubt or problem, whether it's their GP, a helpline or a home care nurse.

Organizing medication treatment is another priority. Managing medication at home can be complex, especially if the patient has to take several medications at different times of the day. The caregiver must therefore ensure that the patient fully understands his or her prescription, explaining the reason for each drug, how and when to take it, and the importance of not interrupting treatment without medical advice. The use of weekly pillboxes can be encouraged to make it easier to organize doses. It is also important to inform the patient and those close to him/her of the potential side-effects of medication, and of signs that would require a doctor to be contacted, such as abnormal bleeding under anticoagulants, or a drop in blood pressure under beta-blockers. Finally, the caregiver can remind patients of the importance of follow-up appointments to adjust treatments if necessary.

Monitoring for signs of relapse or complications at home is an integral part of post-hospitalization counseling. The patient must be able to recognize symptoms that require immediate medical attention. For example, for a patient who has suffered a heart attack or is suffering from heart failure, it is essential to monitor signs such as worsening shortness of breath, chest pain, rapid weight gain or the appearance of edema. The caregiver can give the patient a guide with symptoms to watch out for, as well as actions to take in an emergency, such as contacting the emergency services or calling the doctor. This helps reduce the anxiety associated with the fear of not knowing how to recognize a complication, and helps empower the patient to take responsibility for managing his or her own health.

Adapting the home environment is often necessary to facilitate recovery at home, especially for patients with physical limitations after prolonged hospitalization. The caregiver can advise on the layout of the home to make daily life safer and more comfortable. For example, it may be advisable to secure carpets or slippery surfaces, install grab bars in the bathroom, or raise beds or chairs to facilitate sit-to-stand transitions. For patients who need to limit physical effort, the caregiver may advise centralizing activities in a single room, or limiting the number of times they go up and down stairs. These adjustments reduce the risk of falls or excessive fatigue, and allow the patient to concentrate on recovery.

Managing physical activity at home is another important aspect of post-hospitalization advice. Even moderate physical activity plays a key role in recovery, improving blood circulation, strengthening muscles and preventing complications such as thrombosis. However, it is essential that exercise is adapted to the patient's abilities and state of health. The caregiver must remind the patient of the importance of keeping moving, while respecting his or her limits. He or she can recommend simple exercises, such as daily walking or light stretching, encouraging the patient to gradually increase the duration and intensity as tolerated. The caregiver can also point out warning signs during exercise, such as severe breathlessness, chest pain or dizziness, and encourage the patient to stop and consult a doctor if these symptoms appear.

Diet and lifestyle management play an essential role in preventing relapses and stabilizing health after returning home. The caregiver can advise the patient on a balanced diet, particularly for patients with heart disease or diabetes. It is often necessary to follow a low-sodium diet to avoid fluid retention, or to reduce consumption of saturated fats to improve cholesterol.

The caregiver can provide practical advice on implementing these dietary changes, such as learning to read food labels, favoring steaming or baking, and increasing consumption of fruit, vegetables and lean proteins. It's also important to remind the patient of the importance of staying well hydrated, unless medically contraindicated. Finally, lifestyle habits such as stopping smoking and reducing alcohol consumption should be discussed, as they play a fundamental role in preventing cardiac complications.

Family support and the involvement of loved ones are also key aspects in ensuring a smooth return home. The caregiver can encourage relatives to get involved in the patient's care, particularly by informing them about the practical aspects of treatment and care at home. This includes advice on how to support the patient in his or her treatment, accompany him or her on physical exercise, or monitor certain clinical signs. It is also important to involve the family in decisions concerning the adaptation of the home environment, in order to facilitate the patient's daily life. The caregiver can also direct relatives to resources or home support services if outside help is needed.

Finally, **the management of follow-up appointments** and continuity of care are crucial to the patient's return home. The caregiver must ensure that the patient knows the dates of his or her post-hospitalization appointments, and has all the information needed to organize them. This includes consultations with the attending physician, check-ups (blood tests, ultrasound scans, etc.), and physical or cardiac rehabilitation sessions. Regular follow-up enables treatment to be adjusted if necessary, and recovery to be monitored. The caregiver can also remind the patient of the importance of noting down any questions or symptoms he or she may wish to raise during these consultations.

Chapter 5

Continuing Professional Development for Cardiology Nurses

Continuing education and training

○ Cardiology training programs for nurses' aides
Cardiology training programs for healthcare assistants play an essential role in improving the skills and knowledge needed to provide quality care for patients with cardiovascular disease. Cardiology is a complex specialty, encompassing a wide range of specific pathologies, treatments and management. As key members of the healthcare team, carers need to be well-trained to understand the basics of cardiac conditions, common procedures, as well as post-operative and rehabilitative care, in order to effectively support patients through their care journey. This training enables caregivers to acquire not only technical skills, but also an in-depth understanding of the human and emotional aspects of caring for cardiac patients.

Cardiac pathology training is one of the main components of cardiology training programs for healthcare assistants. Understanding the various cardiovascular diseases is fundamental to providing appropriate care. Training courses generally include modules on common pathologies such as heart failure, angina pectoris, myocardial infarction, and arrhythmias such as atrial fibrillation. Caregivers learn to recognize the symptoms associated with these conditions, such as shortness of breath, chest pain, edema or palpitations, so they can react quickly and appropriately if the patient's condition deteriorates. This enables him to work closely with nurses and doctors to monitor patients on a daily basis and report any signs of complication.

Learning clinical monitoring techniques is another essential aspect of training programs. Cardiac orderlies must be able to monitor certain vital parameters in cardiac patients, including heart rate, blood pressure, oxygen saturation, and sometimes weight. These measurements are crucial for monitoring the patient's progress, especially for those suffering from heart failure or who are post-operative after cardiac surgery. The training courses include practical exercises in which caregivers learn how to use measuring devices (blood pressure meters, oximeters, etc.)

correctly, and how to interpret results so as to detect early abnormalities. They are also trained to understand the importance of recording these data in care records, and of informing the nursing team of any worrying signs.

The management of post-operative care and medical devices is another key component of cardiology training. After cardiac surgery, patients require specialized care to ensure a good recovery. Caregivers need to be trained in the management of patients who have undergone procedures such as coronary bypass surgery, angioplasty or stenting. This includes monitoring surgical wounds, managing chest drains and preventing infections. In addition, orderlies are often responsible for the management of medical devices, such as central venous catheters, pacemakers or implantable cardioverter defibrillators (ICDs). They need to understand how these devices work, know how to handle them safely, and be able to monitor for any signs of malfunction or infection around the implantation site.

Cardiopulmonary resuscitation (CPR) techniques are also an integral part of training programs for cardiac care assistants. In the hospital environment, where patients are often at risk of sudden complications, it is vital that all nursing staff, including orderlies, are able to react quickly in the event of cardiac arrest. Training courses include practical modules on CPR, the use of automatic external defibrillators (AEDs) and emergency management. These skills enable caregivers to intervene effectively while awaiting the arrival of the medical team, thereby increasing patients' chances of survival in the event of a heart attack.

Rehabilitation care and helping patients to resume physical activity are another important aspect of training. Cardiac patients, particularly those who have suffered a heart attack or undergone surgery, often need to undergo a rehabilitation program to regain their physical condition and improve their quality of life. Caregivers play a key role in this rehabilitation phase, encouraging patients to gradually resume physical activity suited to their condition. Training courses teach them how to monitor patients' reactions to exertion, adapt exercises to their abilities, and help them regain self-confidence. It also includes practical advice on the importance of exercise in strengthening the heart and preventing future complications.

Therapeutic education and communication with patients are also at the heart of our training courses. Caregivers need to be able to explain to patients the importance of following their treatment, complying with medical recommendations and recognizing the warning signs of a complication. This includes the ability to communicate clearly and empathetically, answering patients' questions and allaying their concerns. Training courses emphasize pedagogy and psychology, so that caregivers can support patients in understanding their illness and managing their condition on a day-to-day basis, particularly during the transition from hospital to home.

Finally, **the prevention of complications and nosocomial infections** is one of the essential skills taught in these training programs. Cardiac patients, especially those confined to bed or wearing medical devices, are particularly vulnerable to infection. Caregivers learn to follow strict hygiene protocols, handle medical devices with care, and watch for signs of infection (redness, warmth, discharge, etc.). Pressure sore prevention and thrombosis monitoring are also part of this training, as prolonged immobilization can lead to serious complications.

- ◦ Certifications and specializations available

The certifications and specializations available to healthcare assistants represent important opportunities to enrich their skills, deepen their expertise in a specific field, and thus offer more specialized, higher-quality care. In cardiology as in other medical specialties, these certifications enable caregivers to train in the latest techniques and acquire cutting-edge knowledge, while distinguishing themselves within their profession. The healthcare field is evolving rapidly, and specializing not only helps to improve patient care, but also to meet the new demands of the healthcare system. These certifications and specializations are often offered by nursing schools, hospitals or accredited continuing education organizations.

Certification in cardiac care for nursing assistants is one of the most sought-after specializations in the field of cardiology. It provides an in-depth understanding of the most common cardiac pathologies, as well as specific management techniques for patients suffering from cardiovascular disease. This certification covers aspects such as the management of post-operative care, the monitoring of patients after procedures such as angioplasty or bypass surgery, and the prevention of complications such as thrombosis and edema. It also includes in-depth training in the management of medical devices used in cardiology, such as pacemakers, implanted defibrillators and catheters. This knowledge enables caregivers to work effectively in specialized cardiology departments, where constant and precise monitoring of patients' vital signs is essential.

Specialization in cardiac rehabilitation is another important certification, particularly for caregivers who wish to focus on the recovery phase of patients after a major cardiac event. This training teaches them to coach patients in the gradual resumption of physical activity and to support them in managing the lifestyle changes necessary for their recovery. Cardiac rehabilitation includes therapeutic education skills, where the caregiver learns to explain to the patient the importance of physical exercise, balanced diet and stress management to avoid relapse. This type of certification gives caregivers the tools they need to guide patients through their recovery journey, ensuring they comply with medical instructions and adopt a healthier lifestyle.

Certification in palliative care is a particularly valuable specialization for caregivers working with patients at the end of life, especially in intensive care units or cardiology. Certification in palliative care provides caregivers with training in pain management, emotional support and end-of-life care management. It enables them to develop specific skills for accompanying patients and their families through difficult times, ensuring that the patient's last days are as comfortable and dignified as possible. This specialization includes modules on empathic communication, active listening and managing the psychological aspects associated with the end of life, skills that are essential for providing sensitive, humane care.

Specialization in geriatrics is particularly useful for caregivers working with elderly patients suffering from cardiovascular disease or other chronic conditions. The aging population is often faced with complex problems, combining cardiac disorders with other age-related pathologies, such as loss of autonomy or cognitive impairment. This specialization gives caregivers additional skills to manage the care of the elderly, taking into account the specificities linked to the aging of the body and the increased vulnerability to chronic diseases. They learn to assess the needs of elderly patients, monitor signs of complications and implement strategies to prevent falls, undernutrition and infections.

Certification in cardiopulmonary resuscitation (CPR) techniques and defibrillation is an essential skill for all healthcare assistants, particularly those working in cardiology or intensive care units. This certification enables them to acquire the skills needed to react quickly and effectively in the event of cardiac arrest. Training covers basic cardiopulmonary resuscitation techniques, the use of automated external defibrillators (AEDs), and the management of cardiac emergencies in the critical first minutes before the arrival of the medical team. This skill is essential, as it enables caregivers to intervene immediately in emergency situations, thereby increasing patients' chances of survival.

Specialization in wound care is an important certification for caregivers working with surgical patients or those suffering from chronic wounds, such as those related to poor circulation or heart failure. This training provides specialized skills in wound management, dressings and infection prevention techniques. Caregivers trained in wound healing learn to monitor the progress of surgical wounds, prevent bedsores in bedridden patients, and identify signs of infection or complications linked to poor healing. This is particularly important in cardiology wards, where healing after surgery is crucial to the patient's recovery.

Certification in the prevention and management of nosocomial infections is another relevant specialization for healthcare assistants working in high-risk hospital environments. Nosocomial infections represent a major danger for hospitalized patients, especially those undergoing invasive procedures or debilitated by chronic pathologies. This certification trains orderlies in infection prevention techniques, the use of personal protective equipment (PPE), and the management of asepsis protocols to minimize the risk of contamination. They also learn to identify the first signs of infection, such as fever or redness around medical devices, and to react quickly to prevent the spread of these infections.

Certifications in mental health and psychological support are also important specializations, as they enable caregivers to better understand and manage the psychological aspects of care. In cardiology, patients often face high levels of stress, anxiety and, sometimes, depression, especially after traumatic events such as a heart attack or cardiac surgery. Caregivers specializing in psychological support learn to listen empathetically, spot signs of emotional distress and collaborate with psychologists or psychiatrists to ensure comprehensive care. They play an important role in supporting patients beyond their physical needs, taking into account their mental and emotional health.

- ○ Participation in specialized conferences and seminars

Attending specialized conferences and seminars is an invaluable opportunity for caregivers, particularly those working in cardiology or other medical specialties, to enrich their knowledge, acquire new skills and keep abreast of advances in their field. These events offer a privileged forum for exchanging ideas with experts, researchers and practitioners from a variety of disciplines, while helping to develop a professional network that can prove invaluable in day-to-day practice. By taking part in these meetings, caregivers reinforce their expertise and bring more innovative and effective practices to their care teams.

Specialized conferences and seminars are first and foremost places for continuing education, where healthcare professionals can deepen their understanding of diseases, treatments and care techniques. In cardiology, for example, these events provide an opportunity to learn about the latest advances in the treatment of cardiovascular disease, the management of complications or the use of new medical devices. For caregivers, taking part in such conferences enriches their knowledge of cardiac pathologies, gives them a better understanding of patient management strategies and enables them to improve their day-to-day practices. At these events, they can attend presentations on a variety of topics, such as post-operative care management, monitoring techniques for patients on anticoagulant therapy, or modern approaches to cardiac rehabilitation. These presentations, often led by recognized experts, offer up-to-date information based on the latest medical research.

The practical dimension of specialized seminars is another plus for caregivers. In addition to theoretical presentations, many seminars offer practical workshops, where participants can practice new care techniques or the use of medical equipment. For example, a workshop on cardiopulmonary resuscitation (CPR) and the use of defibrillators enables caregivers to hone their skills in these vital areas, increasing their ability to respond effectively in an emergency. Similarly, workshops on the management of medical devices, such as pacemakers or central venous catheters, offer concrete training that can be immediately applied in daily practice. These interactive sessions, often led by experienced trainers, enable participants to acquire new know-how while receiving personalized feedback on the techniques they have learned.

Attending conferences is also an opportunity to discover innovations in healthcare. The healthcare sector, and cardiology in particular, is constantly evolving thanks to technological advances and medical breakthroughs. New monitoring tools, more efficient medical devices and more effective care protocols are regularly presented at these events. Caregivers attending these conferences are therefore exposed to emerging technologies, such as remote monitoring devices or digital tools for patient data management. By better understanding these innovations, they can not only improve their practices, but also play an active role in implementing them within their teams. As intermediaries close to patients, they can also provide valuable feedback on the use of these technologies in day-to-day care, helping to adapt them to patients' needs.

Specialized conferences and seminars are also a great opportunity for caregivers to exchange ideas with their peers and network with healthcare professionals from other facilities or regions. The informal exchanges that take place at these events - in coffee breaks, round tables or discussion sessions - enable practical experiences, challenges and solutions to be shared. These interactions are a source of inspiration and mutual enrichment. For example, an orderly working in the cardiology department of a hospital can talk to another professional about effective strategies for motivating patients to undergo cardiac rehabilitation. These exchanges encourage the dissemination of best practices and reinforce the feeling of belonging to a community of caregivers sharing the same objectives: improving the quality of care and support for patients.

Attending specialized seminars can also open up career and professional development prospects. By attending conferences, caregivers can discover specialization paths that are of particular interest to them, such as cardiac rehabilitation, palliative care in cardiology, or cardiovascular disease prevention. These events often provide an opportunity to meet trainers, training managers or experts in these fields, who can direct caregivers towards continuing education programs or specialized certifications. What's more, taking part in these events is a way of being recognized as a professional committed to progress and improvement, which can open up opportunities for advancement within the institution or in innovative research or care projects.

The impact of conferences on the quality of care is undeniable. When caregivers attend seminars and conferences, they bring back new ideas and practices to share with their colleagues. This enables them to develop practices within their departments, improve patient care and better respond to the day-to-day challenges encountered in care. For example, after attending a conference on the prevention of nosocomial infections, an orderly may suggest new methods of disinfection or management of medical devices, which can reduce the risk of infection in vulnerable patients. This dissemination of acquired knowledge benefits not only the caregiver, but the entire care team and, by extension, patients.

In addition, **specialized conferences enable caregivers to enhance their communication and presentation skills.** Some seminars offer participants the opportunity to present case studies, care improvement projects or initiatives carried out in their facility. This not only enables them to share concrete experiences with other professionals, but also to develop their communication, organization and project management skills. These presentations are also a way for caregivers to actively contribute to the evolution of care practices and demonstrate their commitment to quality care.

Last but not least, **participation in these events fosters a continuous learning mindset**. By stepping outside their usual practice environment, care assistants are exposed to new ideas, varied perspectives and different approaches to care. This encourages them to adopt an open attitude to change, and to continue learning throughout their careers - an essential aspect in a field like healthcare, where knowledge and technology are constantly evolving. This helps to reinforce their professionalism and their ability to offer care that is ever more adapted to their patients' needs.

Stress and emotional management

◦   Stress management strategies in hospitals

Stress management in the hospital environment is a crucial issue for healthcare professionals, and particularly for orderlies who are at the heart of day-to-day care. Working in a hospital environment can be particularly demanding, due to the emotional burden, the fast pace, the management of emergencies and the pressure of caring for often vulnerable patients. Ineffective stress management can not only affect caregivers' well-being, but also the quality of the care they provide. It is therefore essential to implement appropriate strategies to help caregivers manage stress and preserve their mental health, while maintaining a high level of professional performance. These strategies, which combine personal, organizational and relational approaches, aim to prevent burnout, build resilience and promote a more serene working environment.

Managing time and priorities is one of the first essential strategies for reducing stress in the hospital environment. The pace of work can be intense, with multiple tasks to complete within a limited timeframe, and caregivers can easily feel overwhelmed. To avoid burnout, it's crucial to learn how to organize your days effectively, by setting clear priorities. One method is to identify urgent and important tasks, while delegating or postponing less pressing ones. This makes it easier to manage moments of overload and keep control of your workload. Using simple tools, such as to-do lists or tracking charts, helps you to structure yourself and avoid the accumulation of small unfinished tasks, which can become an additional source of stress.

Effective communication with the healthcare team is another key strategy for reducing stress in the hospital environment. Working in a hospital environment requires constant coordination between team members, and communication problems can quickly lead to misunderstandings, mistakes and increased tension. Caregivers therefore need to develop assertive communication skills to express their needs, ask for help when necessary, and share important information with their colleagues. For example, when the workload becomes too heavy, or complex situations require the intervention of a nurse or doctor, the caregiver must be able to quickly point out these needs without fear of appearing incompetent. Clear, regular exchanges with the team help to better distribute tasks and avoid feelings of isolation or overload.

Day-to-day relaxation and stress management techniques play a crucial role in helping caregivers maintain emotional balance in the face of the challenges of hospital work. Among these techniques, deep breathing and mindfulness meditation are particularly effective in reducing anxiety and regaining a state of calm, even in the middle of the working day. These practices enable you to release accumulated tension, refocus and regain mental energy. For example, during a break, the caregiver can practice abdominal breathing by inhaling deeply for a few seconds, then exhaling slowly, to lower the heart rate and release stress. Mindfulness meditation, which consists in concentrating fully on the present moment without judgment, can also be practiced even in a hospital environment, simply by paying attention to sensations, breathing or the immediate environment. These moments of refocusing, however brief, can relieve some of the stress and allow you to return to the task in hand in a more relaxed state.

Social support and solidarity between colleagues are also decisive factors in managing stress in the hospital environment. Feeling part of a team and sharing experiences with colleagues helps to reduce feelings of isolation, which are often exacerbated during periods of intense stress. Creating a caring work environment, where everyone supports each other, makes it easier to cope with day-to-day difficulties. For example, a buddy system or support system between caregivers can be set up, enabling each member of the team to benefit from a sympathetic ear in times of need, or to have someone to rely on during more difficult times. These positive interactions strengthen team cohesion and help to manage tense situations more effectively.

Managing emotions and maintaining professional distance are essential skills for preventing emotional exhaustion. Working in a hospital environment involves daily contact with suffering patients, which can have an emotional impact on caregivers. It is therefore important to strike the right balance between the empathy needed to support patients and the ability not to be overwhelmed by their emotions. Caregivers must learn to recognize their own emotional limits and accept that, despite their best efforts, certain aspects of the disease are beyond their control. This does not mean being indifferent, but rather knowing how to maintain a professional distance so as not to be constantly absorbed by the emotional burden of patients. In the event of a particularly difficult situation, such as a death or traumatic event, it is essential to be able to talk about it with a colleague, psychologist or supervisor, to prevent these emotions accumulating and becoming a source of prolonged stress.

Work-life balance is also fundamental to stress management. Caregivers, often faced with demanding work schedules and long on-call periods, need to ensure that they have time for rest and disconnection outside of work. It's important to make time for activities that recharge the batteries and take the pressure off, whether they're physical activities, creative hobbies or time spent with family and friends. The idea is to be able to refocus on oneself and recuperate mentally and physically, so as to return to work with renewed energy. Rest periods must be respected, and it's essential not to sacrifice your personal life for work, as this can lead to burnout in the long term.

Ongoing training and the acquisition of new skills can also contribute to better stress management. Uncertainty or lack of confidence in one's ability to cope with complex situations can increase feelings of stress. Taking part in specialized training courses can reinforce skills, enable you to learn new care techniques and better master clinical aspects, thereby boosting self-confidence and reducing anxiety when faced with delicate situations. What's more, continuing to learn and develop brings a sense of accomplishment and self-esteem, which in turn makes it easier to cope with everyday challenges.

Finally, **psychological resources and institutional support** are essential for stress management. Many healthcare establishments offer psychological support programs or group sessions to help professionals cope with daily pressures. It's important that caregivers feel free to access these resources without stigma. Regular sessions with a psychologist can provide a safe space for expressing difficulties and obtaining tools to better manage stressful situations. Hospitals can also organize stress management workshops, discussion groups or group relaxation sessions to promote well-being in the workplace.

       ◦   The importance of peer support and supervision

Colleague support and supervision play a fundamental role in the well-being of caregivers and the quality of patient care, particularly in a hospital environment where pressure and stress are often high. Teamwork, mutual support and supervision provide a framework of security, solidarity and sharing, enabling caregivers to cope better with everyday challenges, learn continuously and prevent burnout. These aspects of professional life create a more humane working environment, where everyone feels supported, valued and able to progress, both professionally and personally.

Colleague support is essential for a number of reasons. In a hospital environment, where situations can be unpredictable and days busy, it's essential to be able to count on colleagues to manage moments of work overload, stress or emotional difficulty. Working in a climate of solidarity not only makes you feel less isolated, but also enables you to learn from each other, share experiences and develop common strategies for dealing with complex situations. Where there is mutual support, tasks can be better distributed, tense moments better managed, and mistakes potentially avoided. For example, a colleague may come to the aid of another caregiver who is overwhelmed by the number of patients to be cared for, or share practical advice on how to resolve a difficult situation.

This **cooperative dynamic** also promotes the smooth flow of care. By working together, caregivers can better coordinate patient care, ensure that tasks are carried out rigorously, and cover needs more effectively. Support among colleagues means they feel more secure in the decisions they have to make, because everyone knows they can count on the others to validate an action or propose an alternative solution. This builds trust within the team and reduces the feeling of individual pressure.

On an emotional level, support from colleagues helps to manage the most difficult aspects of the job, particularly situations of suffering, death or psychological distress among patients. These can be very trying times for caregivers, who are often on the front line when it comes to accompanying patients in moments of great vulnerability. Being able to share their feelings with colleagues, express their emotions without being judged, and find reassurance within the team is crucial to avoiding the build-up of emotional tensions. For example, after a particularly stressful event, such as a death or emergency, a simple conversation with a colleague can relieve some of the stress and prevent it from building up.

Supervision plays an equally important role in guiding and supporting caregivers. It provides a structured framework in which caregivers can learn, ask questions and receive feedback on their work. Supervision, often provided by referring nurses or healthcare managers, is essential to ensure that care is delivered in line with protocols and good practice, while providing a space for dialogue and reflection to improve professional skills.

The role of supervision is twofold: educational and protective. From an educational point of view, supervision provides caregivers with a supportive environment in which they can ask questions about complex procedures, seek clarification on certain aspects of care, or receive advice on how to better organize their work. This support helps reinforce technical skills and boost self-confidence. For example, a first-time caregiver can be coached during his or her first delicate interventions, such as managing a patient on a catheter or in intensive care. Supervision ensures that everything is done correctly, while providing a safe learning environment.

On the protective side, **supervision helps prevent errors** and ensures patient safety. By regularly supervising the work of caregivers, referents can ensure that protocols are followed, care practices comply with standards, and caregivers comply with safety instructions. This is particularly important in departments where care is complex, such as cardiology or intensive care. Supervision provides a safety net for caregivers who, while being responsible for their actions, benefit from additional expertise to validate or correct their actions.

Supervision also provides an opportunity to reflect on professional practice. During supervision sessions, care assistants can discuss situations encountered, reflect on decisions taken, and analyze the results obtained. This enables continuous improvement in care practices, taking into account feedback and suggestions from supervisors. This continuous improvement approach is essential for developing skills, identifying weak points and reinforcing good practices. For example, after a patient complication, a supervision session can provide an opportunity to look back on the event, identify what could have been done differently, and draw lessons for the future.

Colleague support and supervision also help to prevent burn-out, a common risk among caregivers due to the demanding and emotionally taxing nature of their work. Knowing that you're not carrying the load alone, that you can count on colleagues when you need them, and that you benefit from structured support helps to alleviate stress and better manage accumulated fatigue. Constant support allows you to share difficult moments, relieve emotional pressure and avoid isolation, which is one of the major factors in burn-out.

Finally, **recognition by peers and supervisors** is essential to boost motivation and self-esteem. In a hospital environment, where the pace of work is often intense and the days long, receiving encouragement, thanks or positive feedback on one's work is extremely motivating. Whether it's a colleague acknowledging a job well done, or a supervisor recognizing the professionalism of a care assistant, such recognition boosts self-confidence and gives meaning to daily work. Knowing that one's work is appreciated and useful within the team contributes to a sense of job satisfaction.

  ◦   Relaxation and recovery techniques

Relaxation and recovery techniques are essential for caregivers, especially in demanding environments such as hospitals, where stress, emotional load and physical fatigue can quickly accumulate. Self-care is a necessity for maintaining good mental and physical health, preventing burnout and continuing to provide quality care. These techniques, which encompass a variety of approaches, enable caregivers to release tension, restore energy and better manage the daily demands of their profession. Learning to integrate moments of relaxation and recuperation into the daily routine can make a significant difference to overall well-being.

Deep breathing and cardiac coherence are accessible and effective relaxation techniques, particularly suited to caregivers looking for quick ways to manage stress during the day. Deep breathing, also known as diaphragmatic breathing, involves taking long, slow inhalations, followed by prolonged exhalations. This calms the nervous system, slows the heart rate and reduces accumulated tension. A few minutes of conscious breathing, particularly during a break or between treatments, can be enough to restore a sense of calm and reduce anxiety. Cardiac coherence, which involves synchronizing breathing with a regular rhythm (for example, five seconds of inhalation followed by five seconds of exhalation), has also been shown to reduce stress and improve concentration.

Mindfulness meditation is another relaxation technique that is gaining in popularity in the healthcare sector. Mindfulness involves concentrating on the present moment, observing sensations, thoughts and emotions without judgment. For care assistants, often overwhelmed by emergencies and pressure, practicing mindfulness helps them to step back from stressful events and avoid being drawn into anxious ruminations or anticipations. A few minutes of mindfulness, even during a break, can help you refocus and take a mental break in a sometimes chaotic environment. This can include simple awareness of body sensations or breathing, or careful observation of the immediate environment, such as the sound of ambient noise or the texture of an object.

Stretching and progressive muscle relaxation are particularly beneficial for caregivers, who are often confronted with physical pain due to prolonged postures, patient handling or repetitive movements. Regular stretching throughout the day helps release muscular tension and improve blood circulation. For example, stretching the back, shoulders and legs helps reduce aches and prevent back pain, which is common in the care professions. Progressive muscle relaxation involves successively contracting and releasing each muscle group, starting with the feet and working up to the head. This technique enables you to become aware of areas of tension in the body and gradually release them, inducing a sensation of deep relaxation.

Moderate physical activity is another effective means of recovery, not only releasing tension but also stimulating the production of endorphins, the feel-good hormones. Walking, cycling or swimming are all accessible activities that help to disconnect from daily stress while improving physical fitness. For caregivers, the regular integration of even light physical activity is crucial to maintaining a good balance between the mental workload and physical recovery. Physical exercise also helps to improve sleep, which is often disrupted among caregivers due to irregular working hours or night shifts.

Yoga and tai chi are practices that combine relaxation, movement and breathing, and are particularly beneficial for carers. These disciplines promote deep relaxation while improving flexibility, muscle strength and balance. Yoga, for example, with its gentle postures and breathing exercises, helps to release accumulated tension in the body while calming the mind. Certain postures, such as those that open the chest or stretch the back, are particularly recommended for caregivers, who spend long hours standing or bending over. Tai chi, with its slow, flowing movements, helps strengthen concentration and calm the nervous system. These practices can be incorporated at the end of the day to promote complete recovery after a period of intense work.

Digital disconnection and moments of silence are also important recovery techniques, especially in a world where the omnipresence of screens and constant solicitations can exacerbate stress. For caregivers, who are often faced with sensory overload in the hospital environment, allowing themselves moments without phones, computers and notifications is essential to regaining a form of mental calm. Silence and disconnection help to rest the brain, reduce constant stimulation and encourage reflection or simply soothing. This can take the form of a few minutes away from noisy spaces, or a screen-free evening at home to allow genuine relaxation.

Restorative sleep remains one of the key elements of recovery, but it can be disrupted by the irregular schedules of caregivers. It is therefore essential to implement strategies to promote quality sleep, even when nights are short or fragmented. This can include establishing a regular sleep routine, trying to go to bed and get up at the same time whenever possible. It's also important to create an environment conducive to sleep: a dark, quiet, cool bedroom, and avoiding screens for at least an hour before bedtime. If you find it difficult to fall asleep, relaxation techniques such as meditation or deep breathing can be used to calm the mind and make it easier to fall asleep.

Finally, **conscious breaks** during the day are another necessary form of recuperation to avoid the accumulation of fatigue. In hospital environments, it can be tempting to skip breaks or reduce them to a minimum because of the workload. Yet taking real breaks, even short ones, can help you recover mentally and physically, and improve productivity in the long term. These breaks can be used to take a short walk, breathe deeply, drink water or simply sit down in a quiet place to release the pressure. They are essential for maintaining sustained attention and avoiding errors due to fatigue.

Career prospects and development opportunities

◦ Career opportunities in cardiology
The field of cardiology offers many opportunities for caregivers who wish to broaden their skills, deepen their knowledge and take on more responsibility within their career. This medical sector is both complex and constantly evolving, with technological advances, new treatments and increasingly personalized approaches to patient care. Caregivers who take this path can not only enhance their expertise, but also access a wide range of professional opportunities, from specialization to care coordination, and even training and management functions.

Specialization in cardiac care is one of the first career options for cardiac care assistants. Working in a specialized department, such as a cardiac intensive care unit or cardiac rehabilitation unit, requires specific training to master the particularities of caring for patients with cardiac pathologies. These patients often require increased monitoring and complex management of their care, involving mastery of medical devices such as cardiac monitors, catheters and defibrillators. Specializing in these areas enables the caregiver to become an expert in technical care, and to assume greater responsibility in the management of critically ill or recovering patients.

Cardiac rehabilitation is another career path for cardiology nurses. After a heart attack or surgery, patients need close support to resume appropriate physical activity, manage their diet and modify their lifestyle habits. Caregivers who specialize in cardiac rehabilitation play a key role in this crucial phase of recovery. By undergoing additional training, they can support patients as they gradually regain their independence, supervising exercise programs and educating them about preventive behaviors to avoid further complications. This rehabilitation work is rewarding, as it enables us to follow patients over the long term and see first-hand the positive impact of the care provided.

Cardiology care coordination is another career path for experienced orderlies. With experience and specific training in care management, an orderly can move into a coordinating role within a cardiology department. This role involves ensuring continuity and fluidity of care between the different members of the medical team, ensuring good communication between nurses, doctors and other healthcare professionals, and guaranteeing that patient care complies with protocols and quality standards. Care coordination also includes logistical management, such as organizing care schedules and priorities, as well as administrative follow-up. This type of position requires organizational, leadership and communication skills, while remaining close to the care teams.

Ongoing training and mentoring are also potential career paths for cardiology orderlies. With experience, an orderly can become a trainer or supervisor for new generations of carers. As a referent in his or her department, he or she can help new caregivers learn specific cardiology care techniques, pass on technical knowledge and offer support in complex situations. Supervision also includes the possibility of contributing to the development and implementation of care protocols, organizing ongoing training sessions for the whole team, and participating in the improvement of care practices within the hospital. This move towards teaching responsibilities enables you to enhance your expertise, while having a lasting impact on the quality of care provided in your department.

Cardiology research also offers an interesting career path for nursing assistants with a passion for innovation and improving practices. By training in clinical research methodology, caregivers can take part in research projects within their healthcare establishment, particularly in the context of clinical trials on new cardiology treatments or devices. They can contribute to the development of evidence-based care protocols and participate in the dissemination of research findings into clinical practice. Involvement in research enables them to remain at the cutting edge of advances in cardiology, and to play an active role in the evolution of the nursing profession.

International opportunities are another possibility for cardiology orderlies. Many healthcare establishments abroad are looking for healthcare assistants qualified in specific fields, such as cardiology. By acquiring recognized expertise in this field, an orderly can consider working in other countries or taking part in international exchange programs. These experiences enable them to enrich their skills by discovering other healthcare systems, other care practices and new approaches to treating cardiovascular disease. It also helps develop language and cultural skills, while offering a broader perspective on the challenges of global health.

Finally, **specialization in cardiac palliative care** is another option for caregivers wishing to focus on supporting patients at the end of life or suffering from terminal heart failure. Palliative care in cardiology requires particular sensitivity, as it involves both technical management of symptoms, such as breathlessness or pain, and human accompaniment, to help patients and their families through this difficult stage. By specializing in this field, caregivers can play a crucial role in improving patients' quality of life at the end of the course, while offering psychological and emotional support.

○   Expanded roles and greater responsibility

In the care sector, and particularly in cardiology, healthcare assistants can take on expanded roles and increased responsibility, as they gain experience and train in more specialized skills. The evolution of their role reflects a general trend in the healthcare sector, where front-line caregivers, such as orderlies, are playing an increasingly crucial role in the overall care of patients. This rise in responsibility is accompanied by a recognition of their expertise and their importance in the organization of care. Thanks to ongoing training and growing confidence on the part of the medical team, nursing assistants are able to evolve towards positions involving greater autonomy and leadership.

One aspect of these expanded roles is the more active involvement of orderlies in the clinical monitoring of patients, particularly in specialist departments such as cardiology. Thanks to an in-depth knowledge of cardiac pathologies acquired through experience and training, orderlies can be tasked with monitoring critical vital parameters such as blood pressure, heart rate or oxygen saturation. By closely observing these indicators and rapidly identifying abnormalities, they play an essential role in preventing complications, particularly in post-operative patients or those on anticoagulant therapy. The responsibility of pointing out early warning signs of complications or deterioration in clinical condition enables caregivers to make an active contribution to patient safety.

Technical care management is another area in which nursing assistants may find their responsibilities increasing. For example, in cardiac intensive care units, they are often required to handle complex medical devices under the supervision of the nursing or medical team. These devices include catheters, pacemakers and cardiac monitors, all of which require rigorous attention. Caregivers trained in these technical practices may be involved in the management and maintenance of such equipment, ensuring that it functions properly and that safety procedures are followed. This increased responsibility demands technical precision and constant monitoring, reinforcing the key role of caregivers in specialized care.

Taking on more autonomous responsibility for certain aspects of daily care is another sign of the increasing responsibility of orderlies. With experience, an orderly can be expected to manage basic but critical patient care independently. This may include managing hygiene care for patients wearing medical devices, administering care to cardiac rehabilitation patients, or helping bedridden patients mobilize. Autonomy in taking on these tasks not only relieves the nursing teams, but also ensures more personalized and attentive patient follow-up. With greater responsibility, the caregiver becomes a key player in the overall monitoring of patients' health, ensuring that care is delivered with consistency and quality.

Therapeutic education is another area in which caregivers can see their role evolve. Cardiac patients often need specific support to help them understand their disease, follow their treatment and adopt best practices to avoid complications. In this context, caregivers trained in therapeutic education can play an active role in informing patients about the day-to-day management of their disease. For example, they can explain how to monitor their blood pressure or weight, adjust their diet to better control cardiac risks, or encourage them to engage in appropriate physical activity. This educational responsibility strengthens patient autonomy, while ensuring better adherence to treatment.

Involvement in care improvement projects and inter-professional collaboration are other areas in which care assistants can play a greater role. In healthcare establishments, it is becoming increasingly common to see care assistants involved in working groups or committees concerned with improving care practices. Their practical expertise and proximity to patients give them a unique perspective on the real needs of patients and the challenges encountered in delivering day-to-day care. Participating in these initiatives enables caregivers to propose concrete solutions to improve the quality of care, whether by optimizing protocols, improving coordination between teams or proposing new methods to enhance patient well-being.

Managing communication with families is also an important responsibility that caregivers can take on as part of their wider role. In cardiology, where patients and their families can face stressful and complex situations, communication with families is paramount. Through their daily contact with patients, orderlies are often on the front line in answering families' questions, reassuring them and providing them with information on their loved ones' state of health. By taking charge of some of this communication, under the supervision of doctors and nurses, caregivers help maintain an essential link between the nursing team and patients' loved ones, contributing to a more humane and serene care environment.

Supervisory and managerial roles are also available to experienced orderlies. Over time, an orderly may move into a supervisory or managerial role, where he or she will be responsible for training new recruits, supervising their practices and ensuring that standards of care are met within the department. This role involves imparting technical knowledge, encouraging the autonomy of new caregivers while guiding them, and ensuring that the care provided complies with the facility's protocols and expectations. This represents recognition of the expertise accumulated over the years, and a step towards managerial responsibilities while remaining close to the heart of the nursing profession.

Finally, **nursing assistants may also be entrusted with responsibilities in team** and schedule **management**, particularly in departments where the organization of care is complex, such as cardiology. Managing schedules, distributing tasks and coordinating care between the various members of the nursing team are all crucial aspects in ensuring the smooth running of a hospital department. Experienced care assistants, with their detailed knowledge of patient needs and the capabilities of their colleagues, can be called upon to play a role in this organization, ensuring that care is well planned and that human resources are optimized to meet the demands of the department.

In conclusion, **nursing assistants have the opportunity to see their roles broaden and take on increased responsibilities over the course of their careers,** particularly in specialized departments such as cardiology. Thanks to ongoing training, acquired experience and close collaboration with medical teams, they can become key players in patient monitoring, technical care management, therapeutic education and communication with families. This move towards greater autonomy and responsibility reflects the growing importance of their role within the healthcare team, and their ability to make a significant contribution to the quality of care provided.

- ○ The importance of involvement in clinical research and practice improvement projects

Involvement in clinical research and practice improvement projects is of crucial importance for caregivers, particularly in specialized fields such as cardiology. Not only does it contribute to the evolution of care and the continuous improvement of practices, but it also enhances the skills and expertise of caregivers, while actively involving them in innovation and the optimization of care quality. By getting involved in these initiatives, care assistants not only deliver care according to current standards, they also actively participate in their evolution, and become agents of change in the healthcare system.

Involvement in clinical research puts caregivers at the heart of medical and technological advances. In cardiology, where treatments and devices are evolving rapidly, clinical research plays a fundamental role in developing new therapies, improving surgical techniques and managing complex cardiac pathologies. Participating in clinical research means that caregivers work with multidisciplinary teams to test new protocols, evaluate the efficacy of experimental treatments and contribute to data collection. This active participation in research ensures that the care provided is based on the best available scientific evidence, thereby improving patient safety and treatment efficacy. For example, as part of a clinical trial involving new anticoagulants or cardiac monitoring devices, caregivers can contribute to the close monitoring of patients, the collection of clinical data, and the monitoring of side effects, working in close collaboration with researchers and doctors.

Involvement in these projects also promotes a better understanding of diseases and treatments, as it enables caregivers to acquire more in-depth knowledge of pathological processes and therapeutic innovations. This knowledge enriches their day-to-day practice, enabling them to better understand the reasons for the interventions or treatments prescribed to patients. By being at the heart of clinical research, nursing assistants become valuable information relays within their teams, sharing the latest discoveries with their colleagues and contributing to the dissemination of evidence-based practices. This strengthens their role within the care team, and makes them key players in the implementation of new practices.

Projects for improving practices, or continuous improvement in the quality of care, are just as essential to the evolution of care. In the hospital environment, caregivers are the first to witness the needs, problems and potential improvements in patient care. They are therefore particularly well placed to identify areas where changes can be beneficial, whether to optimize care efficiency, improve patient comfort or enhance safety. By taking part in practice improvement projects, orderlies become key players in adapting protocols, evaluating procedures and innovating care management. For example, in a cardiology unit, an improvement project could aim to reduce complications linked to nosocomial infections, improve patient management after surgery, or optimize monitoring of heart failure patients at home. Caregivers can make an essential contribution by proposing concrete modifications to care protocols based on their practical experience.

These practice improvement projects also enable us to respond more effectively to patients' needs, and to adapt care based on their feedback. Listening to patients and their families, combined with careful observation by care assistants, helps to identify areas for improvement in the care provided. For example, a project may aim to better organize communication between the care team and patients' families, or to improve therapeutic education for patients so that they better understand their treatments and adopt behaviors conducive to their recovery. Involving caregivers in this type of approach helps to make care more humane and personalized, taking into account the specific needs and expectations of each patient.

Involvement in clinical research and practice improvement projects also enhances caregivers' professional fulfillment. Participating in these initiatives enables them to step outside the confines of routine tasks and get involved in projects that have a direct impact on the quality of care. This brings a sense of accomplishment and contribution to the greater goal of constantly improving the healthcare system. What's more, these experiences enrich caregivers' professional careers, as they develop new skills in project management, data analysis, communication and teaching. They become essential resources within their establishments, able to initiate and lead innovation projects while continuing to provide front-line care.

Involvement in these initiatives also strengthens interdisciplinary collaboration. Clinical research and practice improvement projects are not the concern of a single profession, but are based on cooperation between nursing assistants, nurses, doctors, researchers and care managers. By working together, these professionals bring complementary perspectives that enrich our thinking and enable us to propose more appropriate and effective solutions. Caregivers, through their direct, daily contact with patients, play a key role in this collaboration, providing invaluable information on the reality of care and contributing to the practical implementation of proposed changes.

Last but not least, **our involvement in clinical research and the improvement of practices helps to advance the entire nursing profession**. Every innovation, every successful project contributes to enhancing the role of nursing assistants in the medical team and demonstrating the added value of their expertise. This strengthens recognition of their work, and paves the way for greater responsibility and autonomy. What's more, by taking part in these projects, caregivers can share their results with other establishments or at conferences, thus contributing to the development of practices on a wider scale and the dissemination of best practices.

Chapter 6

Technology and Innovations in Cardiology

Technological tools for caregivers

○ Introduction to monitoring technologies: Holter, portable ECGs, etc.

The introduction of cardiology monitoring technologies, such as Holter, wearable ECGs and other connected devices, has revolutionized the way cardiac patients are monitored and managed, both in hospital and at home. These tools enable continuous and more accurate monitoring of cardiac activity, offering better detection of abnormalities, more proactive management of pathologies and optimization of patient treatment. For caregivers and other healthcare professionals, it is essential to understand the use and benefits of these technologies, as they not only improve the quality of care, but also help prevent complications and tailor treatments to each patient's specific needs.

The cardiac Holter is one of the most commonly used technologies in cardiology for continuous monitoring of cardiac activity. It is a portable device that records a patient's electrocardiogram (ECG) over a period of 24 hours, or even longer. Unlike a standard ECG, which only captures a snapshot of cardiac activity, the Holter enables heart rhythm to be monitored over an extended period, which is crucial for detecting intermittent abnormalities, such as arrhythmias, that might not show up on a traditional ECG. This device is particularly useful for patients who experience palpitations, dizziness, or other occasional cardiac symptoms that might not be observed during a conventional consultation.

For nurses, understanding how the Holter works is important, as they are often involved in installing it on patients and monitoring its correct use on a daily basis. The Holter consists of electrodes placed on the patient's chest, connected to a portable device. Once the device has been installed, the caregiver must ensure that the electrodes are correctly positioned, and that the patient is comfortable wearing the device for the duration of the recording. They must also explain to the patient how to use the device correctly, particularly with regard to activities to be avoided (such as showering), and how to report times when symptoms are experienced so that these can be correlated with the data collected. The role of caregivers is therefore essential in ensuring that the data collected by the Holter is of the highest quality, and can help doctors to make an accurate diagnosis.

Wearable ECGs, often in the form of small connected devices or even smartphone accessories, are another major innovation in cardiac patient monitoring. These devices enable patients themselves to perform electrocardiograms autonomously, in just a few seconds, when they experience unusual symptoms, such as palpitations or chest pain. In addition to the 12-lead ECG, which is performed in hospital, portable ECGs enable more reactive and immediate monitoring of cardiac events. Results can then be transmitted directly to the doctor via an app, facilitating rapid management if an abnormality is detected.

The use of portable ECGs requires caregivers to make patients aware of their correct use. Indeed, although these devices are designed to be simple to use, it is important that the patient understands when and how to use them. Caregivers can also play a key role in training patients, explaining how to position the electrodes or sensors, how to interpret the device's warning signals, and how to transmit results to the medical team. They ensure that patients are comfortable with this technology, especially the elderly or those less at ease with digital tools.

Ambulatory blood pressure monitors, used to monitor blood pressure over 24 hours, represent another key technology for the management of cardiovascular pathologies. These devices are particularly useful for diagnosing masked or resistant hypertension, which may go undetected during standard consultations. The monitor records blood pressure variations throughout the day and night, providing a more precise view of the patient's blood pressure fluctuations. This makes it possible to fine-tune antihypertensive treatments or prevent complications such as stroke or heart failure.

Once again, caregivers play an important role in installing and explaining the device to the patient. They must ensure that the cuff fits properly, and that the patient understands how the device works, particularly with regard to the frequency of measurements and the activities to be performed or avoided during recording. They can also reassure patients who may feel worried or embarrassed about wearing this type of device for an extended period.

Remote monitoring devices are another technological advance that is transforming cardiac patient monitoring, particularly for those suffering from chronic conditions such as heart failure. These systems make it possible to remotely monitor key parameters such as heart rate, blood pressure, and even oxygen saturation via wearable or implantable devices. These technologies, often connected via apps or digital platforms, give doctors and care teams real-time access to patient data, without the need for systematic hospital visits. This enables more reactive management of high-risk patients, and can prevent unnecessary hospitalization by detecting early signs of cardiac decompensation.

For caregivers, the introduction of telemonitoring represents an opportunity to evolve towards new practices. Their role is often to ensure that patients know how to use these technologies at home, that they understand the importance of data transmission, and that they follow the recommendations for remote monitoring. In addition, caregivers can be involved in the day-to-day monitoring of alerts generated by these systems, helping to detect anomalies early and coordinate the necessary interventions.

The benefits of these monitoring technologies are manifold, for patients and caregivers alike. They enable more personalized care, based on objective, continuous data. Patients benefit from greater autonomy and peace of mind, knowing that they are being proactively monitored. For caregivers, these technologies offer a better understanding of fluctuations in patients' health status, enabling them to react more quickly to problems, adjust treatments in real time, and improve the overall quality of care.

   ○   Use of medical software for patient follow-up
The use of medical software for patient monitoring has become an essential element of modern healthcare management, particularly in cardiology. These technological tools help to improve the efficiency, precision and quality of care by centralizing patient data, improving the coordination of care teams, and optimizing clinical decisions. For caregivers, the integration of this software into their day-to-day work means more rigorous monitoring, rapid access to relevant information, and an active role in managing the patient's care pathway.

Centralizing medical information is one of the key benefits of patient monitoring software. Instead of handling paper files that can be difficult to consult and update, medical software centralizes all patient health data on a digital platform. This includes medical history, test results, diagnoses, current treatments, and notes from various consultations. This centralization gives caregivers rapid access to the information they need to provide the right care for each patient. For example, when a patient enters a cardiology unit, the caregiver can, thanks to medical software, immediately consult his or her cardiac history, previous examinations such as ECGs or cardiac echograms, and current treatments. This enables better preparation of care and greater reactivity in case of need.

Treatment and care management is another area where medical software offers real added value. These tools make it possible to keep precise track of the drugs administered, the doses prescribed and the times at which they are taken, thus avoiding errors and oversights. In pathologies such as heart failure, where patients are often required to take medications at specific times (such as diuretics, beta-blockers or anticoagulants), managing treatments via medical software enables real-time monitoring of medication administration and prevention of drug interactions. Caregivers can

147

consult this information directly, ensuring that each patient receives the right treatment at the right time. What's more, the software often features alert systems to warn of missed doses or deviations in administration, enabling caregivers to quickly rectify the situation.

Monitoring vital signs is also simplified thanks to these digital tools. Medical software enables real-time monitoring and recording of vital patient data, such as blood pressure, heart rate, oxygen saturation or temperature. This information is entered directly into the software, often via connected devices, and provides a global and continuous view of the evolution of the patient's state of health. For caregivers, this facilitates daily monitoring of patients, particularly those at high risk of cardiac complications. They can quickly identify abnormal variations in vital constants and alert the medical team if necessary. For example, a sudden rise in blood pressure or drop in oxygen saturation can be reported immediately, enabling rapid, preventive intervention.

Care planning and coordination also benefit greatly from the use of medical software. On a hospital ward, with its large number of care teams and varied tasks, care coordination is essential to avoid errors and oversights. Software can be used to precisely plan care for each patient, assign tasks to different team members, and monitor progress in real time. For example, in a cardiology unit, care assistants can consult their care schedule on the software, which tells them when to carry out specific tasks, such as taking vitals, managing post-operative care, or accompanying patients in rehabilitation. This planning facilitates the organization of work, improves the flow of care, and ensures that each patient receives the care he or she needs at the right time.

Communication between care teams is also facilitated by the use of medical software. These tools enable patient information to be shared in real time between the various players in the care pathway, be they doctors, nurses, care assistants or other healthcare professionals. This is particularly important in departments such as cardiology, where decisions often need to be taken quickly and in a coordinated fashion. For example, when a doctor modifies a treatment or prescribes an additional examination, this information is immediately available to the whole team via the software. Care assistants can therefore adapt their care to the latest medical recommendations without the risk of miscommunication or delays in implementing decisions.

In addition to facilitating communication within healthcare teams, **medical software also enables patients' appointments and examinations to be better tracked**. In the management of chronic pathologies, such as heart failure or coronary disease, patients are often required to undergo regular examinations and follow-up consultations. Software enables these appointments to be managed more efficiently, by scheduling consultations, cardiac ultrasounds or stress tests, and sending automated reminders to caregivers and patients. This ensures that patients don't miss any important tests, and that their follow-up is regular and comprehensive.

The management of discharge files and follow-up at home is also improved thanks to medical software. When a patient leaves hospital after cardiac surgery or hospitalization for an acute pathology, the software enables the preparation of a complete discharge file, containing all information relating to the patient's state of health, the care received and recommendations for follow-up at home. Caregivers play an important role in this transition phase, ensuring that patients and their families understand post-hospitalization instructions. Thanks to medical software, they can easily consult and print out this information, explain it to patients and ensure that everything is clear before discharge.

Last but not least, **medical software ensures enhanced traceability and safety of care**. Every action performed on a patient is recorded in the system, guaranteeing complete traceability of care. This includes not only treatments administered, but also interventions, consultations and examinations. In the event of a problem or dispute, this traceability makes it possible to retrace the history of care and check that all actions have been carried out in accordance with current protocols. For care assistants, this offers additional security, as each treatment is recorded and validated, minimizing the risk of error.

    ◦   The impact of telemedicine on cardiac patient follow-up

The impact of telemedicine on cardiac patient care is considerable, and is profoundly transforming the way care is delivered in the field of cardiology. Thanks to technological advances, telemedicine enables patients to be monitored remotely, chronic diseases to be managed proactively, and home consultations to be offered, all while improving the quality of care and reducing unnecessary hospitalization. For patients with cardiac pathologies, who often require close, continuous monitoring, telemedicine offers a new approach to care, combining accessibility, rapid intervention and personalized treatment.

One of the main benefits of telemedicine in monitoring cardiac patients is the ability to perform continuous remote monitoring of critical cardiac parameters. Thanks to connected devices such as blood pressure monitors, portable electrocardiograms and heart rate sensors, patients can now measure their vital constants at home. These data are then transmitted directly to cardiologists or care teams, who can analyze the results in real time. This continuous monitoring is particularly important for patients with heart failure, atrial fibrillation or high blood pressure, as it enables early detection of signs of decompensation or worsening of the disease, often before the patient experiences significant symptoms.

For caregivers and other healthcare professionals involved in monitoring cardiac patients, **telemedicine facilitates day-to-day care management**, by providing constant visibility of changes in patients' state of health. Caregivers, for example, can be tasked with monitoring alerts generated by connected devices and rapidly contacting patients if any anomalies are detected. This makes it possible to act proactively, by adjusting treatments or offering rapid consultations, before the situation becomes critical. This remote monitoring considerably reduces emergency hospitalizations, which can be avoided thanks to early intervention.

Telemedicine also promotes patient autonomy, enabling them to play an active role in managing their own health. Cardiac patients, who are often frail and require rigorous monitoring, can use telemedicine to measure their blood pressure, heart rate or weight themselves, and transmit the data to their doctor without having to travel. This autonomy is particularly appreciated by elderly patients or those with reduced mobility, for whom frequent trips to the hospital can be tiring. What's more, this approach enables patients to better understand their disease, by visualizing fluctuations in their vital constants themselves, and becoming aware of the impact of their lifestyle on their heart health.

For patients living in rural areas or far from medical centers, **telemedicine reduces inequalities in access to care**. Thanks to remote consultations, patients can benefit from regular follow-up with their cardiologist, without having to travel long distances. This enables close monitoring of chronic diseases, even for patients living in regions with a poor medical infrastructure. This remote monitoring is essential to detect problems early and ensure continuity of care, even at a distance. By making care more accessible, telemedicine improves the equity of the healthcare system, ensuring that all cardiac patients, regardless of where they live, can benefit from quality care.

Online consultations via secure platforms are another aspect of telemedicine that has revolutionized cardiac patient follow-up. Instead of having to visit the hospital for routine check-ups, patients can now consult their cardiologist remotely, via videoconferencing. This enables doctors to assess the patient's state of health, discuss symptoms or treatment side-effects, and make real-time decisions on care management. For patients, this simplifies medical follow-up, while offering the possibility of regular consultations and treatment adjustments without leaving home. What's more, these online consultations enable cardiologists to provide rapid care when needed, without the waiting times often associated with in-office consultations.

Another major impact of telemedicine on cardiac patient monitoring is the increased personalization of care. Thanks to the data continuously collected by connected devices, doctors can better understand patient-specific trends and adapt treatments according to the variations observed. For example, by monitoring heart rate or blood pressure over several weeks, a cardiologist can more precisely adjust medication doses, avoid overdosing, and better anticipate care needs. This personalization of treatment is particularly beneficial for patients suffering from heart failure or complex arrhythmias, where regular adjustment of treatment is often necessary to stabilize the disease. What's more, these data enable us to adopt a more preventive approach, avoiding complications before they arise.

For caregivers, **the use of telemedicine also changes their role in monitoring cardiac patients**, placing them at the center of remote care coordination. Indeed, they may be responsible for liaising between patients and cardiologists, monitoring data transmitted by connected devices, and checking that patients are complying with follow-up recommendations. Caregivers play a key role in educating patients on the use of these technologies, explaining how to use home monitoring devices, how to interpret warning signals, and how to react in the event of anomalies. In addition, their hands-on role with patients ensures that they understand the importance of remote monitoring and their active involvement in managing their disease.

However, integrating telemedicine also requires adjustments to ensure optimal follow-up. Caregivers need to be trained in the use of digital platforms and the management of connected devices to guarantee the quality of remote care. Patients, particularly those who are elderly or unfamiliar with technology, may require initial support to master the use of telemedicine tools. It is therefore essential to offer ongoing support to ensure that all patients can take full advantage of the benefits of telemedicine.

Innovations in cardiology: what caregivers need to know

- New implantable devices: Pacemakers, automatic defibrillators, etc.

New implantable devices, such as pacemakers and implantable cardioverter defibrillators (ICDs), represent major advances in modern cardiology. They offer effective, long-term care for patients suffering from heart rhythm disorders, heart failure and other serious cardiovascular pathologies. Thanks to these technologies, it is now possible to continuously regulate, stimulate and monitor cardiac activity, while considerably reducing the risk of serious complications such as cardiac arrest or life-threatening arrhythmias. These devices, which are becoming increasingly powerful and miniaturized, not only improve patients' quality of life, but also extend their life expectancy by providing constant monitoring and automatic intervention in the event of heart failure.

The pacemaker, one of the best-known and most widely used implantable devices, is designed for patients suffering from bradycardia (slow heartbeat) or heart block. These heart rhythm disorders can lead to dizziness, fainting, or even cardiac arrest in the most severe cases. The pacemaker works by sending regular electrical impulses to stimulate the heart and maintain a normal heart rhythm. This device, implanted under the skin in the chest, is connected to the heart by probes (electrodes) which detect the electrical activity of the heart muscle and send impulses when a slowdown is detected.

153

Modern pacemakers feature advanced functions. They can automatically adjust their rhythm according to the patient's needs, for example by increasing the heart rate during physical exertion or reducing it at rest. This ability to adapt to individual needs enables patients to lead more active lives, and not be limited by variations in their heart rate. In addition to this dynamic regulation, today's pacemakers are equipped with integrated monitoring systems that collect data on heart function and the activity of the device itself. This information can then be transmitted remotely to doctors for ongoing monitoring and possible adaptation of treatment.

The implantable cardioverter defibrillator (ICD), on the other hand, is a device designed to treat serious arrhythmias, such as ventricular tachycardia or ventricular fibrillation, which can lead to sudden cardiac arrest. The ICD, as its name suggests, has the ability to automatically detect dangerous arrhythmias and intervene by sending an electric shock to restore a normal heart rhythm. This device is essential for patients at high risk of cardiac arrest, as it enables immediate intervention in an emergency, where every second counts. Unlike external defibrillators, used in hospitals or by emergency services, the ICD is implanted directly under the skin and operates autonomously, without external intervention.

The latest generation of implantable automatic defibrillators are also equipped with intelligent features. In addition to delivering electric shocks, these devices can also administer gentler pulses to treat certain arrhythmias without the need for a shock. This improves patient comfort, as shocks can be experienced as traumatic. The ICD also monitors cardiac activity in real time and records all data relating to arrhythmia episodes, enabling cardiologists to assess disease progression and better understand the triggers of attacks.

Intelligent implantable devices are also capable of communicating remotely with the medical team, thanks to integrated telemedicine systems. This means that pacemakers and

ICDs can transmit regular information on the patient's state of health, the proper functioning of the device and any cardiac events detected, without the patient having to visit the hospital for frequent check-ups. These devices are equipped with remote monitoring systems that can detect early abnormalities and prevent serious complications before they manifest as symptoms. For caregivers, this offers a considerable advantage in terms of monitoring: orderlies and nurses can receive real-time alerts in the event of malfunctions or critical cardiac episodes, and intervene rapidly if necessary.

One of the challenges for patients with these implantable devices is to **understand and adapt to their daily use**. Although modern pacemakers and ICDs are becoming smaller and more discreet, they still require regular monitoring and vigilance. For example, patients need to be informed of the precautions to be taken regarding exposure to electromagnetic fields, which could interfere with the device's operation. Caregivers and nurses play a key role in patient education, explaining how to care for their device, how to recognize warning signs (such as dizziness or palpitations), and how to react in the event of a problem. This education enables patients to live serenely with their device, and to adopt good practices to ensure its smooth operation.

The move towards leadless implantable devices is another major advance in this field. Leadless pacemakers, for example, are miniaturized devices that can be implanted directly into the heart, without the need for conventional leads connecting the pacemaker to the organ. These pacemakers reduce the risk of infection or complications associated with leads, and the procedure for implanting them is less invasive. What's more, these leadless pacemakers last longer and are easier to monitor, representing a significant advance in terms of patient comfort and safety.

In addition to pacemakers and automatic defibrillators, other implantable devices, such as **pacemakers for heart failure**, are increasingly being used. These devices, known as biventricular pacemakers or cardiac resynchronization devices (CRTs), are designed to help the heart beat more synchronously in patients with advanced heart failure. By simultaneously stimulating both ventricles of the heart, these devices improve the efficiency of each cardiac contraction, thereby reducing heart failure symptoms such as breathlessness and fatigue. As a result, patients can better tolerate physical exertion and regain a better quality of life.

       ○   Innovations in care techniques: cardiac catheterization, robotic surgery

Innovations in cardiology care techniques, such as cardiac catheterization and robotic surgery, represent a veritable revolution in the management of cardiovascular disease. These technological advances enable less invasive, more precise and safer interventions, offering patients shorter recovery times, lower risks of complications and optimized therapeutic outcomes. These innovations have not only transformed the way interventions are performed, but have also expanded treatment options for patients who, in the past, would not have been able to benefit from surgical management due to their medical condition.

Cardiac catheterization is one of the most important techniques in interventional cardiology. It is a minimally invasive procedure used to diagnose and treat a number of cardiac pathologies, including coronary artery disease, valvular heart disease and certain cardiac malformations. Catheterization involves inserting a thin flexible tube, called a catheter, into a blood vessel, usually via the femoral artery (in the groin) or the radial artery (in the wrist). This catheter is then guided to the heart under X-ray control, enabling cardiologists to examine the interior of the coronary arteries, visualize any abnormalities, and intervene directly if necessary.

One of the main advantages of cardiac catheterization is that it can be both a diagnostic tool and a therapeutic procedure. **Coronary angioplasty**, a common catheterization procedure, involves dilating a coronary artery narrowed by atherosclerotic plaque, thereby restoring blood flow to the heart. In many cases, a stent (a small metal prosthesis) is inserted into the artery to maintain the opening and prevent further obstruction. This avoids the need for more extensive surgery, such as coronary artery bypass grafting, while offering comparable results in terms of restoring blood flow. Catheterization is also used for percutaneous valve replacement, an alternative to open-heart surgery to replace a defective heart valve, particularly in elderly or high-risk patients.

For patients, the benefits of cardiac catheterization are numerous. **The minimally invasive nature of the** procedure means less pain, scarring and risk of infection than traditional surgery. What's more, recovery is much faster: patients can usually be discharged from hospital after a short hospital stay and resume their normal activities within a few days. This contrasts sharply with the prolonged recovery times and increased risks associated with open-heart surgery. For caregivers, post-operative follow-up is also simplified, as complications are less frequent and post-operative care is often limited to monitoring the incision and vital vitals.

Robotic surgery represents another major advance in cardiology and cardiac surgery. This innovative technique enables surgeons to perform procedures with unrivalled precision, using robotic arms controlled remotely from a console. One of the best-known systems is the Da Vinci robot, which has been widely used for a variety of cardiac procedures, including mitral valve repairs, coronary bypass surgery, and even the correction of congenital anomalies of the heart. Robotic surgery offers greater precision, as it eliminates the natural tremors of the human hand and enables more delicate, controlled movements.

One of the main advantages of robotic surgery is its ability **to reduce invasiveness**. Unlike traditional cardiac surgery, which often requires a complete opening of the thoracic cavity (sternotomy), robotic surgery is generally performed via small incisions, through which the robotic arms are inserted. This minimizes trauma to the patient, considerably reduces post-operative pain, and reduces the risk of infection or other complications. In addition, patient recovery is significantly faster, with reduced hospital stays and shorter convalescence times.

Another major advantage of robotic surgery is that it enables surgeons to access areas of the heart that are difficult to reach using conventional methods. The high-definition 3D vision offered by robotic systems enables very fine visualization of cardiac structures, facilitating complex interventions. For example, in the case of **valve repairs**, robotic surgery enables damaged valves to be reconstructed with extreme precision, improving the chances of successful intervention and reducing the need for artificial valve prostheses. This is particularly beneficial for younger patients, as preserving the natural valves avoids certain long-term risks associated with prostheses.

The impact of robotic surgery on patients' quality of life is undeniable. In addition to the benefits of reduced scarring and pain, the precision of this technique often improves surgical outcomes. For patients suffering from complex heart disease, robotic surgery offers a less invasive solution that is just as effective as conventional surgical techniques. It also opens up prospects for patients considered inoperable with traditional methods due to their fragility or the complexity of their condition.

Caregivers play a crucial role in the post-operative monitoring of these innovations, whether cardiac catheterization or robotic surgery. Although these techniques reduce the need for prolonged intensive care, they require rigorous monitoring of vital signs and close attention to potential complications, such as incision site infection or internal bleeding. Caregivers ensure that patients recover well, accompanying them in the first few days after surgery, making sure that their recovery goes smoothly. Their role is also essential in educating patients about home care, pain management and precautions to take to avoid complications.

The future of these technologies is promising, with many advances still to come. For example, surgical robots are becoming increasingly sophisticated, with thinner, more agile arms, enabling even more delicate interventions. The development of new catheterization techniques, such as fully percutaneous procedures for heart valve repair, promises to make these interventions accessible to a greater number of patients, even those at high surgical risk. What's more, the growing integration of artificial intelligence into robotic surgery opens the way to even more precise and personalized interventions, where every robot movement could be optimized according to the patient's specific characteristics.

○ Emerging treatments and their implications for care

Emerging therapies in cardiology offer new perspectives for the management of cardiovascular disease, particularly in cases where traditional treatments are limited or insufficient. These new approaches, whether pharmacological therapies, innovative medical devices or biological treatments, are not only transforming the way cardiac pathologies are treated, but also redefining the role of caregivers in managing this care. Integrating these innovations into clinical practice is helping to improve therapeutic outcomes, expand options for high-risk patients, and offer more targeted and personalized treatments.

New drug classes are playing a crucial role in these advances. One of the most promising emerging treatments is the use of SGLT2 (sodium-glucose cotransporter type 2) inhibitors in the treatment of heart failure. Initially developed to treat type 2 diabetes, these drugs have shown significant beneficial effects on reducing hospitalization for heart failure and cardiovascular mortality. They act by improving glucose excretion by the kidneys, but their effects go far beyond controlling blood glucose levels. They also reduce the heart's workload by decreasing sodium and water retention, thereby relieving pressure on the heart's walls. For caregivers, these treatments represent an important development, as they have to monitor not only the evolution of the patient's cardiac function, but also the potential side effects associated with this type of therapy, such as urinary tract infections or dehydration.

At the same time, **PCSK9 inhibitors**, a new class of -lipid lowering drugs, have considerably improved the management of hypercholesterolemia in patients at high cardiovascular risk. These monoclonal antibodies reduce LDL-cholesterol levels (the "bad" cholesterol) much more effectively than statins, especially in patients for whom the latter are insufficient or poorly tolerated. By preventing the degradation of LDL receptors in the liver, these inhibitors enable better elimination of circulating cholesterol, thus reducing the risk of serious cardiac events such as myocardial infarction or stroke. These treatments require special monitoring, as they are administered by subcutaneous injection every two to four weeks, requiring patient education and increased vigilance on the part of caregivers to ensure compliance.

Stem cell treatments and gene therapy are also promising avenues of research in the treatment of cardiovascular disease. These approaches aim to regenerate damaged heart tissue, particularly after a myocardial infarction, where part of the heart muscle dies as a result of lack of oxygen. Cardiac stem cells, or even induced pluripotent stem cells, have the potential to repair necrotic tissue and restore heart function. Clinical trials are still in their early stages, but results are encouraging. Gene therapy, on the other hand, targets specific mutations responsible for certain genetic cardiomyopathies. By injecting corrective genes into heart cells, it is possible to prevent disease progression, or even restore normal cardiac function. These treatments represent a break with traditional therapies, as they aim to treat the underlying causes of disease, rather than its symptoms. For caregivers, the challenge is to closely monitor these patients to observe the long-term effects of these therapies, while keeping an eye on possible immunological or rejection complications.

Innovations in implantable medical devices, such as leadless pacemakers or miniaturized heart pumps, are also changing approaches to care for patients with advanced heart disease. For example, left ventricular support devices (LVADs), which are increasingly used as a temporary or permanent solution for patients with end-stage heart failure, can significantly prolong life, while offering improved quality of life. These devices, implanted in the thorax, assist the pumping function of the left ventricle, enabling the heart to better perfuse the organs. Care of these patients is complex, requiring constant monitoring of vital parameters, management of anticoagulants to prevent thrombosis, and prevention of infections linked to the device's external systems.

Transcatheter heart valves, such as TAVI (Transcatheter Aortic Valve Implantation), are another key innovation in the management of valvular heart disease, particularly in elderly or high-risk patients. Replacing defective aortic valves with prosthetic valves via a simple puncture in the femoral artery (without opening the rib cage) offers a less invasive alternative to open-heart surgery. This enables patients previously considered inoperable to receive effective treatment and considerably improve their life expectancy. For caregivers, accompanying patients who have benefited from these procedures means careful monitoring of post-operative complications such as bleeding, stroke or infection.

The implications of these emerging treatments for care are numerous. Firstly, they require caregivers to adapt their skills. The management of patients undergoing complex treatments, such as biotherapies or implantable devices, requires ongoing training to understand the mechanisms of action of new therapies, the monitoring to be put in place, and specific protocols to prevent complications. In addition, caregivers must play a key role in patient education. Many of these innovative treatments, such as PCSK9 inhibitors or heart pumps, require strict compliance and a good understanding of the daily gestures to adopt to avoid complications. Patient support, through clear explanations and regular monitoring, is therefore essential to guarantee treatment success.

These therapeutic innovations are also changing **the role of caregivers in personalizing care**. With treatments increasingly targeted and adapted to patients' genetic or biological characteristics, it is becoming essential to monitor disease progression on an individualized basis. Caregivers, in direct contact with patients, need to be able to quickly identify signs of response or failure of treatments, as well as potential side effects. This implies more detailed monitoring and close collaboration with medical teams to adjust treatments in real time.

Finally, **emerging treatments in cardiology offer the opportunity to reduce hospitalization and improve patients' quality of life**. Thanks to minimally invasive devices or more effective drug therapies, many patients can now benefit from high-quality care at home or in outpatient facilities, alleviating the burden of long, heavy hospital stays. Caregivers, especially nursing assistants, play an essential role in this transition to more autonomous care, helping patients to manage their treatment at home, monitoring warning signs and intervening rapidly when necessary.

Ethics and responsibility in the use of new technologies

◦ Data confidentiality and patient privacy

Data confidentiality and respect for patient privacy are fundamental principles in the healthcare field, particularly in a context where the use of digital technologies and medical information management tools is constantly expanding. The collection, storage and transmission of patient medical data must be carried out with extreme care to ensure that this sensitive information is protected against unauthorized access, misuse or violation of privacy. Respecting confidentiality is more than just a legal obligation; it represents an essential ethical dimension in the relationship of trust between patient and healthcare professional.

The nature of medical data makes this a particularly sensitive issue. Personal health information includes not only medical history, diagnosis and treatment, but also elements such as genetic data, examination results, psychological or psychiatric consultations, and information relating to patients' private lives. These data are among the most sensitive, as they can reveal intimate aspects of a person's life, affecting not only their physical health, but also their psychological and social well-being. Any breach of confidentiality can have serious consequences for patients, ranging from social stigmatization to discrimination in employment or insurance.

Respect for confidentiality is based on several fundamental principles. First and foremost, healthcare professionals, including orderlies, are bound by medical confidentiality, a legal and ethical obligation that prohibits the disclosure of medical information without the patient's informed consent. This means that all information shared by the patient or observed during his or her care must be protected, and only those directly involved in his or her care must have access to it. For example, when a hospitalized patient shares details of his or her state of health or history with a caregiver, the latter is required not to divulge this information to other colleagues not directly involved in the patient's care, nor to outsiders such as friends or family, without the patient's authorization.

The growing use of digital technologies in medical monitoring has added a complex dimension to privacy management. Electronic medical records (EMRs), telemedicine systems and connected devices make it possible to centralize health data, facilitate sharing between healthcare professionals and improve care coordination. However, these technologies also pose risks in terms of data security. Electronically stored information can be vulnerable to cyber-attacks, unauthorized access or human error in database management. It is therefore essential that healthcare establishments put in place strict protocols to guarantee the security of medical data, including data encryption, the use of strong authentication systems, and limited access to electronic records according to caregivers' roles and responsibilities.

For caregivers, **respecting confidentiality when using digital tools** is crucial. For example, when accessing patient information via medical software or monitoring applications, they must ensure that they do so in a secure environment, and that only authorized persons can view the data. It is also important to ensure that computer screens or documents containing medical information are not left visible to unauthorized persons, and to disconnect from computer systems after use to prevent unauthorized access. In addition, when transmitting information to other members of the care team, they must ensure that these exchanges take place in secure environments, such as via encrypted platforms or closed meetings.

Informed patient consent is another key aspect of confidentiality and privacy. Before sharing medical information with other healthcare professionals, or using certain technologies for remote monitoring, it is essential that patients are informed of how their data will be used, stored and shared. Patients must be able to give their consent, but also to withdraw it if they so wish. This consent must be explicit and based on a clear understanding of the implications, which often requires caregivers to take the time to explain to patients what is at stake in health data management. For example, in the context of telemedicine or monitoring via connected devices, it is important for patients to know who will have access to their data, how it will be protected and under what conditions it might be shared.

Confidentiality also extends to day-to-day interactions with patients. Conversations about their state of health should take place in spaces where privacy is protected, such as closed rooms or consulting rooms. Discussing a patient's condition in a corridor or public area of the hospital can compromise confidentiality, even if done with good intentions. The same applies to communication with the patient's family and friends: caregivers must take care to obtain the patient's agreement before sharing information with family or friends, except in an emergency situation justifying a waiver of medical confidentiality.

In addition to protecting medical data, **respect for patient privacy extends to their dignity and physical intimacy**. For example, when a caregiver assists a patient with hygiene care, it is essential to respect the patient's privacy by ensuring that this care is carried out in a private environment, where the patient feels comfortable. The caregiver must also always ask the patient's permission before performing any gestures that involve physical contact or uncovering certain parts of the body, in order to preserve the patient's sense of dignity and control over his or her own body.

Data confidentiality and privacy are also at the heart of trust between patient and caregiver. If a patient feels that their personal information is protected and that their privacy is respected, they will be more inclined to share important details about their condition, which is essential for effective care. On the other hand, a breach of confidentiality can have devastating consequences for this relationship of trust and for the quality of care. A patient who feels betrayed or exposed may be reluctant to provide crucial information, which can hinder diagnosis and treatment.

- ○ The caregiver in the face of AI and care automation

The introduction of artificial intelligence (AI) and automation in healthcare, including cardiology, marks a profound change in the way care is organized and delivered. As an essential member of the healthcare team, the caregiver is now confronted with these technologies, which are overturning certain aspects of the profession while opening up new perspectives. Rather than replacing the role of caregivers, AI and automation are transforming the way we work, bringing tools that complement and enhance care while freeing up time for more human tasks. However, this transition requires adaptation, ongoing training and ethical reflection on the place of machines in patient care.

Artificial intelligence in healthcare is already widely used to analyze complex data, make diagnoses, predict complications and optimize treatments. In cardiology, for example, AI is used to analyze electrocardiograms (ECGs) or echocardiogram images with greater precision, enabling subtle abnormalities to be detected or the risk of heart attacks to be predicted. This ability of AI to rapidly process large amounts of data helps healthcare professionals to make more informed decisions and improve patient care.

For caregivers, **AI can alleviate certain administrative or repetitive tasks**. For example, AI systems can be used to manage care schedules, monitor patient vitals in real time via connected devices, or generate automatic alerts when abnormal parameters are detected, such as high blood pressure or abnormal heart rate. This enables caregivers to focus more on human interaction with patients, spending less time on manual data collection or routine tasks. For example, an AI system can continuously monitor oxygen saturation and send an alert if a patient is desaturated, enabling the caregiver to intervene quickly.

Automation in healthcare also includes the use of robots for certain tasks. In modern hospitals, robots can be used to transport medicines, meals or medical equipment, reducing the physical load on caregivers. Some robots can also assist in mobilizing patients, especially those who are bedridden, reducing the risk of injury to caregivers. These automated devices provide invaluable assistance with logistical tasks and facilitate the day-to-day organization of care, while increasing the safety of nursing staff.

However, **AI and automation cannot replace the very essence of the caregiver's profession**, which relies above all on human accompaniment, listening, empathy and personalized attention to patients' needs. Technologies can improve processes and increase care efficiency, but they cannot replicate a caregiver's ability to detect non-verbal signs of distress, provide emotional reassurance or adapt care to each patient's specific situation. The caregiver plays a central role in the human dimension of care, and this component is irreplaceable.

One of the challenges posed by the introduction of AI and automation is adapting to new technologies. Caregivers must learn to master these tools, understand how they work and use them correctly in their day-to-day missions. This requires ongoing training to integrate these innovations into professional practice. For example, managing home telemonitoring systems or coordinating with automated health data collection systems requires specific skills. The appropriation of these tools by caregivers is essential to ensure that they are used effectively and safely.

What's more, **artificial intelligence can play an important role in improving personalized care**. By analyzing a patient's health data over an extended period, AI is able to suggest treatment adjustments or care more tailored to individual needs. This is particularly relevant for patients suffering from chronic illnesses such as heart failure, where AI can help adjust medication doses according to fluctuations in vital parameters. Caregivers, working closely with the medical team, can use these recommendations to better adapt daily care and prevent complications.

However, **the ethics of using AI and automation in care** raise important questions. While these technologies bring undeniable benefits in terms of efficiency and precision, they can also raise concerns about the dehumanization of care. It is essential to strike a balance between the use of technology and the maintenance of human contact in care. The caregiver, as the direct intermediary with the patient, must ensure that AI is used as a support tool, not as a substitute for human interaction. For example, in a telemedicine context where automated systems monitor the patient's vital data, the caregiver must remain present to respond to the patient's emotional needs, provide physical and psychological support, and ensure that technology is perceived as a help, not a barrier.

The impact of automation on work organization is also an important factor to consider. While automation can relieve caregivers of certain tedious tasks, it can also redefine roles within the care team. This could lead to adjustments in responsibilities, with a transition to more complex, human tasks. For example, care assistants could be given a more central role in guiding patients in the use of medical technologies, in health education and in home care management. This evolution towards more technical skills and a more relational role enhances the value of the nursing auxiliary profession, giving it a more rewarding and specialized dimension.

○ The limits of technology in humanized care

Technological advances in healthcare, whether in artificial intelligence, robotics or remote monitoring devices, have profoundly transformed the way care is delivered, improving the accuracy of diagnoses, the effectiveness of treatments, and the management of chronic pathologies. Yet, despite these impressive advances, there are **inherent limits to the use of technology in humanized care**, limits that remind us that the human dimension of care is irreplaceable. The relationship between caregiver and patient relies on essential elements such as empathy, listening and emotional understanding - aspects that technology, however advanced, cannot fully reproduce. These limitations underline the importance of striking a balance between technological efficiency and the need to preserve humanity in care.

Technology cannot replace empathy and active listening, which are at the heart of humanized care. The simple act of listening to a patient, recognizing and understanding his or her pain, anxieties or concerns, is a fundamental aspect of the caregiver-patient relationship. Orderlies and nurses, for example, play a crucial role by being present to offer reassurance, taking the time to chat with patients, answer their questions or reassure them about the uncertainty of their medical situation. Machines and artificial intelligence systems can provide accurate data, but they cannot understand human emotions, nor can they adapt their responses to a patient's emotional needs. In the case of seriously ill or dying patients, the presence of an empathetic caregiver who accompanies the person through this stage of life cannot be replaced by a robot or technology, however sophisticated.

Human interaction also enables a more nuanced approach to care, taking into account non-verbal signals and feelings that technologies are unable to capture. A patient can sometimes express more through body language or facial expressions than through words. An attentive caregiver can detect these signs and adjust his or her behavior or care accordingly, whether by modifying a position to avoid pain or identifying emotional discomfort. Machines, on the other hand, are only programmed to respond to defined parameters and cannot adjust their behavior in such a subtle and intuitive way. So, although AI can detect physiological anomalies through complex algorithms, it can never replace human sensitivity to perceive silent suffering or a need for attention.

The technology also has its limits when it comes to personalizing care, despite its potential for large-scale data processing. Indeed, although artificial intelligence systems are capable of proposing personalized treatment plans based on medical history and test results, they cannot take into account a patient's personal preferences, lifestyle, cultural beliefs or willingness to adopt one treatment rather than another. The caregiver, through direct interaction with the patient, is able to grasp these aspects, adjust care to specific needs and expectations, and find a compromise between medical efficiency and respect for the patient's individuality. For example, an elderly patient may not wish to undergo invasive surgery despite the machine's technical recommendation, preferring palliative care that focuses more on comfort. A caregiver can facilitate this decision by offering emotional support and understanding that technology alone cannot provide.

The risk of dehumanizing care is another major limitation of the massive introduction of technology into care practices. The automation of tasks, such as taking vital signs via connected devices or using robots to assist patient mobility, can lighten the workload for caregivers, but it can also reduce human contact at times when it is needed. A patient who sees only machines to measure blood pressure, monitor oxygen saturation or deliver medication can feel emotionally distant and isolated. Contact with a caregiver, even for simple tasks, can be reassuring, as it allows the patient to feel that they are being cared for by someone capable of interpreting their needs beyond numbers or results. This human contact is particularly important in situations where patients feel vulnerable or anxious about their illness.

What's more, **the emotional complexity of patients is a dimension that technology struggles to understand and address**. Healthcare is not just about physical treatment; it also encompasses the psychological and emotional support that patients expect. Illness, particularly chronic or severe pathologies, profoundly affects an individual's mental state and emotional balance. A machine cannot alleviate a patient's worries about the future, nor can it offer the empathy and understanding they need to cope with their condition. The role of caregivers, and in particular orderlies, is essential in providing this support, listening, responding to anxieties and establishing a bond of trust. This relationship of trust contributes not only to the patient's psychological well-being, but also to their engagement in their own healing process.

Finally, the biases inherent in **AI systems** and medical technology can be another limitation to the application of these tools in truly humanized care. The algorithms underpinning these technologies are often trained on large databases, but these databases are not always representative of patient diversity. Patients from ethnic minorities or with rare pathologies may be under-represented in these databases, leading to misdiagnoses or inappropriate treatment recommendations. In such cases, the clinical intuition and experience of caregivers remain crucial to

170

rectifying or adjusting technological recommendations. Care automation must therefore be considered with caution, and always accompanied by human supervision to avoid these pitfalls.

Chapter 7

Managing complex cases and versatility in cardiology

Management of polypathological patients

- ° Adapting care to patients with co-morbidities: diabetes, renal failure, etc.

Adapting care to patients with co-morbidities, such as diabetes, renal failure or other chronic pathologies, is a major challenge in medical care. These patients require special attention, as the coexistence of several diseases often worsens their overall state of health and makes their treatment more complex. Each pathology can interact with the others, modifying symptoms, potential complications and response to treatment. For caregivers and other healthcare professionals, it is essential to develop a holistic, personalized approach that takes into account not only each disease, but also the interactions between them, to ensure optimal, safe care.

Diabetes and renal failure are two comorbidities frequently encountered in patients, particularly in cardiology departments, where cardiovascular disease is often associated with these metabolic disorders. Diabetes, for example, is not only a chronic disease in its own right, but also significantly increases the risk of cardiovascular disease and renal failure. Indeed, high blood glucose levels cause long-term damage to blood vessels, affecting both heart and kidneys. Care of a diabetic patient with heart failure therefore needs to take into account not only glycemic control, but also the management of heart failure and the prevention of kidney complications.

Managing diabetes in these patients requires rigorous monitoring of blood sugar levels and regular adjustments to treatments. Caregivers play a key role in this process, helping patients monitor their blood sugar levels, administering insulin or other anti-diabetic drugs, and ensuring that diet follows medical recommendations. Nutrition is particularly important for patients with co-morbidities, as the diet needs to be balanced to control blood sugar levels while being adapted to other conditions, such as renal failure, where it may be necessary to limit protein or potassium intake.

Diabetic patients with renal insufficiency require specific adjustments to their treatments, as **reduced renal function** influences the way drugs are metabolized and excreted by the body. For example, some oral antidiabetic drugs, such as metformin, may be contraindicated in severe renal failure, as they increase the risk of lactic acidosis. Caregivers, in collaboration with nurses and doctors, must be alert to these interactions, watch for signs of complications and report any unusual symptoms such as nausea, weakness or abnormal breathing, which could indicate metabolic dysfunction.

Kidney failure itself also complicates the management of cardiovascular disease, as it limits the use of some commonly prescribed heart medications. For example, diuretics, often used to treat heart failure by reducing water retention, must be adjusted according to the kidneys' ability to filter fluids. Inadequate dosage can lead to dehydration or, conversely, fluid overload, thus aggravating heart failure. In addition, patients with chronic renal failure may develop electrolyte imbalances, such as high potassium levels (hyperkalemia), which increase the risk of cardiac arrhythmia. Monitoring these imbalances is essential, and caregivers must be vigilant for symptoms such as muscle weakness or palpitations.

Adapting care to patients with co-morbidities also requires coordinated management of the various medical teams involved. These patients are often followed by several specialists: a cardiologist for their heart failure, a nephrologist for their kidney failure, and a diabetologist for their diabetes. It is therefore essential that medical information flows smoothly between the various players, so that each treatment takes account of all pathologies. Nurses play a crucial role in this coordination, acting as a link between the various specialists and ensuring that daily care takes into account the specific recommendations of each.

Therapeutic patient **education** is another fundamental aspect of adapting care. Patients with co-morbidities often have to manage several treatments themselves, adjust their lifestyle, and monitor various health parameters, which can be extremely complex. It is therefore essential to help them understand their illnesses and treatments. Caregivers, who are in daily contact with patients, are particularly well placed to provide clear explanations and help them acquire the skills they need to take care of themselves. For example, they can explain the importance of regularly monitoring blood sugar levels, taking medication correctly, and adhering to dietary recommendations adapted to their multiple conditions.

Managing the pain and symptoms associated with multiple pathologies is another major challenge for patients with co-morbidities. For example, a diabetic patient with neuropathy may experience foot pain, while a patient with cardiac insufficiency may experience respiratory discomfort linked to pulmonary edema. Distinguishing the symptoms associated with each pathology is crucial to adapting treatments and providing effective relief. Caregivers must be trained to identify these multiple symptoms, report them to medical teams, and contribute to pain management through daily care, such as pressure sore prevention, adapted mobilization, and hygiene management to avoid infections.

Finally, **psychological follow-up** should not be neglected in patients with co-morbidities. The coexistence of several chronic illnesses can lead to emotional distress, anxiety and even depression. The simultaneous management of several treatments, the fear of complications and the physical fatigue associated with pathologies can weigh heavily on patients' morale. As the members of the health-care team closest to patients, nursing auxiliaries have a key role to play in detecting this psychological suffering. They must be able to offer emotional support, listen to patients' concerns, and refer them to psychological help resources if necessary.

　　　　　　 ◦　　Coordination with other specialist departments
Coordination with other specialized services is a fundamental pillar of comprehensive, high-quality patient care, particularly in

a hospital environment where pathologies are often complex and multiple. Interconnecting care between different medical disciplines helps to better meet the patient's overall needs, avoid errors and ensure continuity of care. In this context, the nursing auxiliary plays a central role in this coordination, serving as an essential link between departments and the various professionals involved in the patient's care pathway. This seamless collaboration is crucial to the patient's well-being and the effectiveness of treatment.

The complexity of multidisciplinary care lies in the fact that each specialist department focuses on a particular aspect of the patient's health, but no department works in complete isolation. Take the example of a patient hospitalized for severe heart failure, who also has chronic kidney problems and poorly controlled diabetes. This patient will probably require close cardiological monitoring, as well as regular consultations with a nephrologist to manage the renal failure, and endocrinological monitoring for the diabetes. The role of caregivers, especially nursing assistants, is to ensure that every care, every treatment and every recommendation is implemented harmoniously, while taking into account the specific needs of each department.

The transmission of information between different departments is a crucial element of this coordination. The caregiver, who is often in direct contact with the patient, is a key player in ensuring that information is shared and understood. For example, after a cardiologist has adjusted a treatment for heart failure, it is essential that the nephrologist is informed of the changes, as certain molecules can affect renal function. Similarly, if an anti-diabetic treatment needs to be modified, it's important that the cardiology department knows whether this treatment could interact with cardiovascular drugs. Nurses play their part by passing on information gathered from patients, such as new symptoms or side-effects, and by collaborating with nurses to ensure that all elements are taken into account in the overall medical follow-up.

Multi-disciplinary meetings are a privileged setting for this inter-departmental coordination. These meetings bring together healthcare professionals from different specialties - doctors, nurses, care assistants, physiotherapists, dieticians, psychologists - to discuss patients' progress, their specific needs, and the adjustments to be made to treatments. At these meetings, each professional brings his or her own expertise to the table, and together they draw up an overall care plan that takes into account the many dimensions of the patient's health. By sharing their knowledge of patients' daily lives - their general condition, their physical capabilities, their need for help with everyday tasks - caregivers make a valuable contribution to these discussions. They offer a practical, patient-focused viewpoint, often complementing that of doctors, who can concentrate on the technical aspects of treatment.

Post-hospital care management is another area where coordination between services is essential. When a patient is discharged from hospital after surgery or prolonged hospitalization, a follow-up plan must be put in place to ensure continuity of care at home or in a rehabilitation center. This requires close coordination between the hospital, homecare services, and possibly other specialized facilities. Caregivers are often involved in this transition, ensuring that patients understand discharge instructions, that medication is taken correctly, and that follow-up appointments are arranged with the various specialists. By ensuring a smooth transition between in-patient and out-patient care, caregivers help reduce the risk of relapse or complications once the patient has returned home.

The management of medical devices and complex treatments is another aspect of interdepartmental coordination. Patients with devices such as pacemakers, insulin pumps or catheters require special monitoring and care. These devices often require the intervention of several specialized departments, and nursing assistants play a role in coordinating these interventions. For example, a patient on dialysis for kidney failure may also need cardiological monitoring to ensure that his or her heart is tolerating the treatment. It is therefore crucial that care related to dialysis, pacemaker management and medication adjustment is coordinated to avoid complications. Caregivers need to be trained to monitor these devices, recognize warning signs and inform other team members in the event of a problem.

The involvement of other paramedical professionals - such as physiotherapists, dieticians and psychologists - in patient care also requires good coordination. For example, for a cardiac patient undergoing rehabilitation, collaboration between the cardiologist and the physiotherapist is essential to establish a suitable exercise program. If the patient is also diabetic, the dietician needs to be involved to adjust the diet to control blood sugar levels, while supporting physical rehabilitation. By following up the recommendations of these different professionals on a daily basis, nursing aides ensure that the patient is following his or her overall care plan. They can also provide valuable feedback by observing how the patient reacts to certain exercises or dietary modifications, enabling the care plan to be adjusted if necessary.

Another reason why coordination is essential **is to prevent medication errors**, which is a frequent risk for patients under the care of several departments. Polymedicated patients, especially those with multiple chronic illnesses, may receive prescriptions from different specialists, and it is essential that these treatments are compatible and their administration monitored. Caregivers play a key role in this monitoring, ensuring that patients receive their medication correctly, that there are no harmful interactions between treatments, and that they follow prescriptions rigorously. For example, in the case of a patient taking anticoagulants for a heart condition and also receiving treatment for kidney disease, particular attention must be paid to dosage adjustments to avoid complications such as bleeding or acute renal failure.

Finally, **coordination with social services** and home help structures is essential for patients in vulnerable situations, whether elderly, chronically ill or disabled. Caregivers can point out non-medical needs, such as home adaptation, access to financial aid or assistance with administrative formalities. This coordinating role is crucial in ensuring that patients receive all the services and assistance they need to live safely and independently after hospitalization.

- ∘ Case studies: Examples of complex patient management

Managing complex patients is one of the major challenges that healthcare professionals, including nursing assistants, are regularly faced with. Patients with multiple chronic conditions, co-morbidities or treatment-related complications require a multi-dimensional, coordinated approach. Through practical case examples, it is possible to illustrate how care needs to be adapted, how caregivers can navigate between different patient needs, and how interdisciplinarity and communication between teams play an essential role in the quality of care.

Case study 1: Patient with heart failure, diabetes and renal failure

Let's take the example of Mr. D., a 65-year-old patient hospitalized for acute heart failure, with a history of type 2 diabetes and chronic renal failure. The management of this patient is complex, as each pathology influences the other, requiring extremely rigorous monitoring and care adapted to each situation.

In the first instance, Mr. D's heart failure requires treatment with diuretics to flush out excess fluid and reduce the heart's workload. However, **diuretics must be carefully monitored**, as they can aggravate renal failure, leading to dehydration or electrolyte imbalance, notably hyperkalemia, which is dangerous for the heart. In this context, caregivers must monitor diuresis (the amount of urine produced) on a daily basis, reporting any significant changes and ensuring that patients are not over-hydrated.

Mr. D's diabetes further complicates care management. Blood sugar levels need to be monitored regularly, as high blood sugar levels can not only worsen kidney condition, but also promote water retention, increasing cardiac load. In addition, the patient's diet needs to be adjusted: **limiting carbohydrates for diabetes**, but also restricting sodium and potassium intake due to heart and kidney failure. Caregivers play a key role in administering anti-diabetic medication, monitoring blood sugar levels, and communicating with the dietician to adjust meals.

Coordination between the cardiology, nephrology and endocrinology departments is essential here. Caregivers, who are closest to the patient, ensure that information is shared between the various specialists. They flag up any changes in the patient's condition - for example, rapid weight gain that could indicate fluid retention, or dizziness that could be a sign of electrolyte imbalance - and ensure that every aspect of treatment is adapted to other pathologies. Their role goes beyond technical care: they also provide emotional support for Mr. D., who is faced with managing several chronic illnesses and the anxiety that goes with them.

Case study 2: Elderly patient with stroke, malnutrition and cognitive impairment

Mrs L., aged 78, was admitted after suffering a stroke which left significant after-effects, including partial paralysis of the left side and mild to moderate cognitive impairment. In addition, she suffers from malnutrition due to difficulties in eating, linked to facial paralysis and a loss of appetite common in elderly patients. Her care is multidisciplinary, and requires special attention from the nursing staff.

Mrs L's stroke has given rise to specific needs in terms of rehabilitation and mobilization. The rehabilitation team, comprising physiotherapists and occupational therapists, set up exercises to restore mobility on the affected side. Caregivers, in collaboration with these specialists, assist the patient on a daily basis with gentle exercises, regular repositioning to prevent pressure sores, and support for safe movement.

Mrs L's **cognitive problems** add a further layer of complexity. Her memory is impaired, and she has moments of confusion. This situation calls for a structured environment and care adapted to her abilities. Caregivers must ensure that instructions are repeated clearly, that care is given at fixed times to avoid disorientating the patient, and that simple explanations are given at each stage of care so that she understands what is happening. Patience and empathy are also essential, as cognitive disorders can cause the patient to become agitated or frustrated.

With regard to undernutrition, Mrs L. receives an enriched diet prescribed by the dietician, but has difficulty chewing and swallowing due to her facial paralysis. The caregivers, trained in techniques for managing swallowing disorders, ensure that she is offered foods that are easy to swallow, monitor her food intake and report any weight loss. They must also ensure that she is well hydrated, regularly offering thickened drinks if necessary. Particular attention is paid to mealtimes, when caregivers play an essential role in encouraging the patient to eat in small quantities, at her own pace, while taking care to avoid the risk of a false start.

Case study 3: Palliative care patient with metastatic cancer and chronic pain

Mr P., aged 59, is admitted to a palliative care unit for the management of chronic pain associated with metastatic cancer. The priority in caring for this patient is comfort, pain management and support towards the end of life. Mr. P. also has respiratory problems and is physically very weak.

Pain management is at the heart of our care. Mr. P. receives opioid treatments to relieve his pain, but these need to be adjusted regularly according to how he feels and any side effects observed, such as drowsiness or constipation. Caregivers play a key role in the ongoing assessment of Mr. P.'s pain, using appropriate scales to quantify his discomfort and immediately reporting any changes to the medical team. They also ensure the correct administration of medication and monitor any adverse effects.

In addition to pain management, **palliative care focuses on quality of life**. Mr. P. suffers from great weakness, and the caregivers help him daily to wash, dress and maintain oral hygiene. They ensure that he is positioned comfortably in bed to prevent bedsores and improve his breathing. The caregivers also provide psychological support, as Mr. P. experiences moments of anxiety and fear in the face of the progression of his illness. Listening to his concerns, offering him moments of relaxation, and encouraging his loved ones to be present are all ways of respecting the human dimension of palliative care.

In this context, coordination with other team members, such as doctors, psychologists, pain nurses and members of the mobile palliative care team, is crucial to Mr. P's overall care. Caregivers, by closely observing the patient's reactions, are often at the forefront of detecting changes in his condition or needs.

Interventions in critical situations

       °   Management of cardiac arrest: advanced resuscitation practices

The management of cardiac arrest is an absolute emergency situation, where every second counts to save the patient's life and minimize potential after-effects. Rapid, effective management relies on well-mastered cardiopulmonary resuscitation (CPR) practices and the use of advanced tools that have evolved considerably over the years. In this critical environment, caregivers and other healthcare professionals must work in close coordination to apply standardized protocols while adapting to each specific clinical situation. Advanced life support practices, integrating both manual techniques and technological devices, are designed to maximize the patient's chances of survival, while ensuring optimal management from the moment of arrest through to hospitalization.

The importance of basic cardiopulmonary resuscitation (CPR) is at the heart of cardiac arrest management. When cardiac arrest occurs, the first objective is to restore blood flow and oxygenation to vital organs, particularly the brain. This is achieved by the immediate application of external chest compressions. Effective CPR involves firm, rapid compressions in the middle of the chest, with a frequency of 100 to 120 compressions per minute and a depth of 5 to 6 centimeters in adults. Caregivers, often on the front line, must be able to start these compressions immediately, even before medical reinforcements arrive, in order to maintain perfusion of vital organs.

Another fundamental aspect of basic CPR is **the importance of artificial ventilation**, which delivers oxygen to the patient's lungs. In a hospital setting, oxygen delivery can be achieved via manual ventilation devices, such as the self-filling balloon (or ambu). Caregivers must master this technique to ensure that air enters the lungs correctly without causing hyperventilation or gastric distension, errors which can compromise the effectiveness of chest compressions and increase the risk of complications.

The automated external defibrillator (AED) is a key tool in the advanced management of cardiac arrest, particularly for sudden cardiac arrest caused by ventricular fibrillation or pulseless ventricular tachycardia. These severe arrhythmias prevent the heart from pumping blood efficiently, and defibrillation is often the only method of restoring a normal heart rhythm. Caregivers trained in the use of AEDs can quickly apply the electrodes to the patient's chest, following voice prompts from the device, which analyzes the heart rhythm and delivers a shock if necessary. The time elapsed between cardiac arrest and defibrillation is crucial to survival: every minute of delay reduces the chances of survival by

7-10%. Caregivers' ability to use this device effectively can therefore make the difference between life and death.

Advanced resuscitation practices, implemented by specialized medical teams, complement basic measures. This includes the use of drugs and other interventions to stabilize the patient after the pulse has been restored, or if initial resuscitation efforts fail. Key drugs include adrenaline, administered to increase perfusion of vital organs in the event of prolonged cardiac arrest, and amiodarone, used to treat arrhythmias refractory to defibrillation. Caregivers, although not responsible for administering these drugs, play a crucial role in monitoring the patient's vital parameters and preparing the necessary devices for the medical team.

In addition to chest compressions and defibrillation, **advanced ventilation devices** are sometimes required, particularly for patients who are unable to resume spontaneous breathing. Tracheal intubation secures the airway and ensures adequate ventilation. Although this technique is reserved for specialized doctors or nurses, nursing assistants help to prepare the equipment, ensure the patient's correct position and monitor the tube to prevent accidental displacement, while keeping an eye on the patient's oxygenation.

In a hospital setting, **coordination between the various medical teams** is essential to maximize the chances of success. Each member of the resuscitation team has a precise role, and fluid communication is crucial. Caregivers, as direct assistants, must be able to adapt quickly to the needs of the team: preparing resuscitation equipment, managing oxygen, monitoring vital signs, while following instructions given by the referring physician.

Another aspect of advanced life support is **post-resuscitation monitoring**, which is essential to stabilize the patient once the pulse has been restored. Restoring blood flow is only the first step, and many complications can arise after cardiac arrest.

Patients need to be closely monitored for signs of deterioration, including heart rhythm disturbances, hypoxia-induced brain damage and multivisceral failure. Caregivers play a key role in this post-arrest phase, closely monitoring vital vitals (heart rate, oxygen saturation, blood pressure) and reporting any abnormalities to the medical team.

Therapeutic hypothermia protocols, often used after successful resuscitation, aim to reduce neurological damage by lowering the patient's body temperature. These protocols involve advanced temperature management techniques, such as the use of cooling blankets or cold serum infusions. Caregivers need to be trained in these procedures to ensure that cooling is carried out in a controlled and safe manner, while monitoring for potential side effects such as electrolyte disorders or cold-induced arrhythmias.

Finally, **the psychological and ethical aspects of resuscitation** must not be overlooked. Managing a cardiac arrest is an intense ordeal, both for the medical teams and for the patient's loved ones. Once the situation has stabilized, nurses may be called upon to provide emotional support to families, who may be in a state of shock. It is crucial to explain what has happened in a clear and empathetic way, while accompanying them in the decisions to come, particularly if a therapeutic limitation is envisaged in the event of an unfavorable neurological prognosis.

○　Managing patients in cardiogenic shock

The management of patients in cardiogenic shock is a complex and delicate emergency situation, requiring a rapid, coordinated response to prevent further life-threatening failure. Cardiogenic shock generally occurs following massive myocardial infarction or severe decompensation of heart failure, when the heart becomes unable to pump enough blood to ensure adequate organ perfusion. This leads to a cascade of complications: generalized hypoxia, multivisceral failure, and without prompt intervention, death. Management of cardiogenic shock therefore relies on immediate assessment, intensive hemodynamic support, and often the use of mechanical devices to assist cardiac function.

Diagnosis and immediate recognition of cardiogenic shock are crucial to prompt management. The first signs are often a sudden drop in blood pressure (severe hypotension), associated with signs of poor organ perfusion, such as mental confusion, cold clammy skin, cyanosis, and oliguria (reduced urine production). Dyspnea (difficulty breathing) is also common, as the heart's inability to pump blood properly causes fluid to build up in the lungs, leading to pulmonary edema. As soon as these first signs appear, nurses and other members of the care team must immediately alert the doctors and prepare the patient for intensive care.

Initial management of patients in cardiogenic shock rests on several pillars. Firstly, it is essential to ensure adequate oxygenation of the patient. Oxygen therapy, and even ventilatory assistance via intubation if necessary, is essential to stabilize respiratory function and prevent worsening hypoxia. Nurses play a key role in this phase, ensuring that oxygen is set up, monitoring the patient's oxygen saturation and assisting nurses and doctors in preparing for intubation if required.

Hemodynamic support is then a priority in the management of cardiogenic shock. The heart, being unable to ensure sufficient cardiac output, often requires the use of inotropic drugs to enhance cardiac contraction, such as dobutamine or adrenaline, as well as vasopressors such as noradrenaline to maintain acceptable blood pressure. These drugs are administered under strict supervision, usually by continuous infusion. Caregivers, although not directly involved in the management of complex infusions, carefully monitor vital signs and report any variations in blood pressure, heart rate or oxygen saturation. They also ensure that peripheral venous lines, used for drug infusion, are set up correctly, and monitor the patient's state of consciousness, which may indicate improvement or worsening of cerebral perfusion.

Fluid management is another fundamental aspect of management. Patients in cardiogenic shock are often in a state of fluid overload, notably due to pulmonary edema, but they may also be in a state of relative hypovolemia (lack of circulating blood volume). The balance is therefore delicate: it is sometimes necessary to infuse fluids in moderate quantities to maintain tissue perfusion, while using diuretics to avoid fluid overload which would aggravate pulmonary edema. Caregivers closely monitor the patient's diuresis, reporting any reduction or absence of urine production (oliguria or anuria), which are signs of poor renal perfusion. This monitoring is essential to guide therapeutic adjustments made by the medical team.

The use of mechanical circulatory assistance devices represents a major advance in the management of cardiogenic shock, especially in cases where pharmacological treatments are not sufficient to restore adequate cardiac function. Among these devices, one of the most common is the intra-aortic balloon pump (IABP), which helps reduce the heart's workload by increasing blood flow to the organs during diastole (the heart's relaxation phase). The implantation of more advanced devices, such as left ventricular assist devices (LVADs), provides mechanical support for the heart when it is in serious failure. Caregivers are involved in monitoring patients on these devices, ensuring that the pumps are working properly and that no mechanical or infectious complications arise. Their role is also essential in observing signs of improvement or deterioration in the patient, such as improved peripheral perfusion or changes in pulse quality.

Rapid revascularization, in cases where cardiogenic shock is caused by myocardial infarction, is essential to improve the patient's prognosis. Angioplasty procedures with stenting or, in some cases, coronary bypass surgery, restore blood flow to oxygen-starved areas of the heart. While these procedures are being prepared, caregivers play a key role in stabilizing the patient, preparing the catheterization room and managing pre- and post-procedure care. After successful revascularization, hemodynamic stabilization and complication management must remain a priority.

Close monitoring of the patient in cardiogenic shock is not limited to hemodynamic parameters. It is also crucial to monitor signs of failure in other organs, particularly the kidneys and liver, which are rapidly affected by lack of perfusion. Cardiogenic shock can lead to acute renal failure (ARF), and regular monitoring of electrolytes, as well as renal function, is essential. Nurses help collect samples for blood tests and monitor urine output, a key indicator of renal function. Signs of liver decompensation, such as jaundice or altered consciousness, must also be monitored and reported immediately.

Psychological guidance and emotional support for patients and their families are also important aspects of cardiogenic shock management. This serious medical situation is a source of great anxiety for patients, who may be aware of the seriousness of their condition, and for their families, who have to cope with the uncertainty of the prognosis. Caregivers, thanks to their proximity to patients, are often the first to pick up on these concerns, and play a key role in providing reassurance, explaining procedures in a simple, reassuring way, and maintaining regular contact with the family to keep them informed of developments.

- ○ Palliative care in cardiology: Supporting patients at the end of life

Palliative care in cardiology is a fundamental aspect of care for patients at the end of life, particularly those with advanced and incurable heart disease, such as end-stage heart failure, severe cardiomyopathy or irreversible complications of myocardial infarction. The aim of palliative care is no longer to cure or prolong life at all costs, but to provide patients with comprehensive support aimed at relieving symptoms, preserving their dignity and improving the quality of their final moments as much as possible. The palliative approach focuses on comfort, taking into account the patient's physical, emotional, social and spiritual dimensions, while actively including the family in the support process.

Managing physical symptoms is one of the primary challenges of palliative cardiology care. Patients with advanced heart failure, for example, often suffer from severe symptoms such as dyspnea (difficulty breathing), edema (fluid accumulation in tissues), and intense fatigue. Dyspnea, a particularly distressing symptom for patients at the end of life, can be managed with palliative treatments such as oxygen therapy to improve breathing, low-dose morphine to reduce the sensation of breathlessness, and diuretics to eliminate excess fluid. Caregivers play an essential role in this phase, monitoring the patient's breathing, adjusting oxygen devices and ensuring overall comfort.

In addition to dyspnea, **pain is another priority in palliative care**. Patients with terminal heart disease may suffer from chest pain or angina pectoris. Pain relief involves the use of opioids, often in combination with other analgesics. Caregivers, in direct contact with patients, must be trained to regularly assess pain intensity using specific scales, and to adapt care to minimize physical discomfort. They also monitor the side effects of drug treatments, such as excessive drowsiness or constipation, ensuring that the patient's overall well-being is maintained.

Emotional and psychological support for palliative care patients is another fundamental aspect of the palliative approach. The end of life is a period marked by profound anxieties, particularly in the face of uncertainty, pain or death itself. Patients with advanced heart disease may also be faced with a sense of progressive decline, loss of autonomy, and dependence on others, which can lead to feelings of frustration, sadness or helplessness. Caregivers, through their constant presence, are often the first to pick up on these emotions, and their role is to offer attentive listening, address the patient's concerns and create a serene, reassuring environment. Regular, even informal, exchanges help to reduce fears and restore a degree of inner peace.

Emotional support is not limited to the patient. **Family support** is a key component of palliative care in cardiology. Loved ones are often faced with difficult emotional dilemmas, such as accepting the approach of death or preparing for the loss of a loved one. They may also experience uncertainty or guilt about decisions made regarding care. In this context, caregivers play a mediating role, facilitating communication between the medical team and the family, explaining treatments and answering relatives' questions. They also help to create a climate conducive to the expression of emotions, offering moments of intimacy between patient and family, while supporting loved ones in their anticipated grieving process.

Consideration of the patient's **spiritual needs** is another essential aspect of palliative care. For some patients, the end of life is a time of deep reflection on the meaning of life, death and what may follow. Spiritual needs can vary considerably from one individual to another, ranging from the need for religious comfort to a more philosophical quest for meaning. Caregivers, while respecting individual beliefs and wishes, can facilitate access to appropriate spiritual support, whether through the presence of a chaplain, moments of prayer or simply respectful, empathetic discussions. This spiritual dimension is crucial to providing comprehensive care, as it touches on the patient's intimacy and his or her way of approaching the end of life.

Managing palliative care in cardiology requires an interdisciplinary approach, where every member of the care team - doctors, nurses, caregivers, psychologists, and spiritual care providers - collaborates to meet the patient's needs. This collaboration ensures that all aspects of care are covered, from physical symptom management to psychological and spiritual aspects. By being in daily contact with patients, caregivers are often invaluable observers, able to detect subtle changes in the patient's physical or emotional state and report these observations to the medical team. Their role goes beyond technical care: they also provide human support, through simple but essential gestures such as adjusting a blanket, offering a glass of water, or simply staying by the patient's side at difficult moments.

In situations where the prognosis is particularly bleak, **ethical decisions concerning the end of life** must be taken in collaboration with the patient, family and medical team. This may involve discussing the cessation of invasive treatments, the limitation of intensive care, or the establishment of advance directives. These decisions, often complex and fraught with emotional consequences, require a sensitive, caring approach. Caregivers, through their close relationship with the patient and family, can help facilitate these discussions by providing emotional support and ensuring smooth communication between all those involved.

Finally, **patient dignity** is a fundamental value that must be at the heart of palliative care in cardiology. It is essential to ensure that every gesture, every decision, is made with respect for the individual, his or her choices, beliefs and life history. This means, for example, respecting the patient's rhythm, avoiding unnecessary interventions that could prolong suffering without any real benefit, and ensuring that care focuses on comfort and quality of life. Caregivers, by being close to the patient in these intimate moments, play a key role in preserving this dignity, through the gentleness of their gestures, their attention to detail and their ability to adapt care to individual needs.

Versatility : Adapt to different contexts

○ Work in different types of units (USC, intensive care, emergency, etc.)

Working in different types of unit, such as the Continuing Care Unit (CCU), the Intensive Care Unit (ICU) or the Emergency Department (ED), requires great flexibility, specific expertise and the ability to adapt to the unique needs of each environment. Each unit has its own dynamic, clinical and organizational specificities, as well as distinct requirements in terms of patient care. Caregivers, as key members of the care teams, play a fundamental role in these diverse environments. They have to adapt their approach to the characteristics of each unit, while ensuring continuity of quality care and meeting the varied needs of patients in often critical situations.

Working in a Continuing Care Unit (CCU) requires constant vigilance and enhanced monitoring of patients who, although stabilized after a critical phase, still require close follow-up. These patients may be discharged from intensive care, but still require close monitoring, notably because of the severity of their condition or the risk of complications. In the ICU, nursing assistants play an essential role in supporting patients during this transitional phase. Their job is to regularly monitor vital parameters (such as heart rate, blood pressure or oxygen saturation), observe signs of deteriorating clinical condition and immediately report any abnormalities to the medical team. Caregivers must also manage specific devices, such as catheters, drains or probes, while ensuring that hygiene, nutrition and comfort care are provided in a safe and respectful environment.

In the USC, patients are often recovering from complex surgery or an acute medical episode, such as a heart attack. **Supporting patients towards progressive autonomy** is an integral part of the caregivers' work. They help patients to regain their motor skills and resume simple activities, such as walking or eating independently, while keeping an eye on them to prevent falls or other accidents. This support is crucial in preparing patients for their return to a conventional unit or home.

The intensive care unit (ICU), on the other hand, is an environment marked by high intensity and constant monitoring. Here, patients are often in critical condition and require advanced life support, with devices such as respirators, circulatory support devices and complex cardiac monitors. Caregivers working in this unit need to be comfortable using this equipment and have a clear understanding of the vital signs to be monitored, as the slightest change can indicate a rapid change in the patient's condition. For example, a change in respiratory rate or a drop in oxygen saturation could require immediate intervention.

In intensive care, **multidisciplinary teamwork** is particularly crucial. Each professional has a defined role, but all must work in a highly coordinated way to ensure patient safety. Caregivers, in this context, are the eyes and ears of nurses and doctors: they spend most of their time at the patient's bedside, and are often the first to detect subtle changes in the patient's condition. They must therefore be able to communicate effectively with the nursing team, report precise observations and play an active role in monitoring complex treatments.

Emergency departments, on the other hand, are characterized by a wide variety of clinical cases and a fast pace of work. Every patient arriving in the ER can present a very different clinical picture: from the elderly with an acute respiratory infection, to the victim of a road accident, to a heart attack or a minor injury. Emergency care assistants must therefore be extremely versatile, able to move quickly from one situation to another and deal with the unexpected. **Patient reception and initial triage** are often tasks in which they are involved, assisting the nurse in the rapid assessment of vital signs and determining the degree of urgency of each situation. This requires a high level of responsiveness and the ability to remain calm under pressure, as decisions taken in the emergency department can have immediate consequences for the patient's survival.

In the emergency departmentorderlies , may be called upon to manage primary care, such as applying dressings, assisting with immobilization techniques for fractures, or helping to resuscitate a patient in cardiac arrest. Their role is crucial in supporting the continuous flow of patients and enabling medical teams to concentrate on critical interventions. **Managing stress and emotion** is an important aspect of emergency work. Faced with sometimes traumatic or highly urgent situations, orderlies need to keep their cool and stay focused, while also being able to offer psychological support to patients and their families in moments of extreme anxiety.

In the intensive care unit, where patients are in critical condition and often on life-support, caregivers are also on the front line. Patients in this unit, often intubated and ventilated, require complex technical care and constant monitoring. As well as providing hygiene and comfort care, orderlies are also involved in the management of medical devices. They ensure correct positioning of the patient to avoid pressure sores, provide regular mobilization to prevent complications linked to prolonged bed rest, and monitor signs of deterioration. Communication with the patient, even under sedation, remains essential: talking to the patient, informing him/her of the procedures performed and maintaining a human relationship helps to preserve his/her dignity and provide comfort, even in an altered state of consciousness.

In all these types of unit, **the ability to adapt** is one of the most valuable qualities of nursing assistants. Each unit has its own pace, its own requirements and its own challenges. Working in such varied environments demands flexibility, a mastery of technical gestures and a keen sense of observation. Caregivers must also know how to adapt to the different tools of communication and coordination within multidisciplinary teams. The transmission of information is essential, whether during team changes or exchanges with doctors. Their responsiveness, keen observation of clinical signs, and ability to manage emergency or crisis situations make them essential players in patient care, whatever the department in which they work.

> ° Management of interdepartmental and interhospital transfers

The management of interdepartmental and interhospital transfers is an essential component of inpatient care, particularly in cases where the patient's condition requires specialized expertise or equipment not available in the original department or hospital.

Transfers, whether internal or external, must be carried out with absolute rigor and seamless coordination between all the teams involved. For caregivers, this process implies not only well-oiled logistics, but also attentive accompaniment of the patient throughout the transfer, in optimum conditions of safety and comfort.

Interdepartmental transfers within the same establishment are often necessary when a patient's condition changes, requiring care in a unit better suited to his or her clinical condition. For example, a patient hospitalized in general medicine may be transferred to intensive care if his or her condition deteriorates, or conversely, a patient initially admitted to intensive care may be transferred to a continuing care unit (CCU) when stabilized. This type of transfer requires careful assessment of the patient's condition, logistical preparation and good communication between the different departments.

Coordination between medical teams is essential in this type of transfer. First and foremost, doctors from the two departments concerned consult each other to define the patient's clinical needs, the reasons for the transfer and the future care arrangements. Caregivers, for their part, play a key role in preparing the patient. This includes checking that all medical devices are functional and ready for transport (e.g. infusions, catheters or drains), stabilizing the patient prior to transfer, and preparing an up-to-date medical record for transmission to the new department.

Patient safety during transfer is an absolute priority. It is essential that all the equipment needed to maintain the patient's stability is available and ready to use in the event of an emergency. Caregivers, in collaboration with nurses, ensure that the patient's vital signs are closely monitored throughout the process. If the patient is on respiratory assistance, infusion or any other complex medical device, they ensure that these systems operate continuously throughout the transfer. Care must be taken when mobilizing patients, especially those with injuries or delicate devices.

Inter-hospital transfer, on the other hand, is often more complex, and occurs when the patient requires care that cannot be provided in the facility where he or she is initially cared for. This may be the case for highly specialized surgical procedures, advanced treatments or access to better-equipped intensive care units in a referral hospital. Inter-hospital transfers are generally organized in emergency or critical situations, making them all the more delicate to manage.

Inter-hospital transfer requires rigorous organization, involving **coordination between two separate establishments**. The medical teams at the sending hospital must first obtain the agreement of the receiving hospital, where a place on the ward must be guaranteed for the patient. This process is followed by the transmission of essential medical information: patient history, diagnosis, current treatments and recent test results. As part of this process, nursing assistants are involved in collecting this information, preparing the patient's medical file and ensuring that all the necessary elements (examinations, biological results, medical imaging) are included.

Medical transport is often required for inter-hospital transfers, especially when the patient's condition is critical. This type of transport can be carried out by ambulance, helicopter or other medical vehicle, depending on the urgency and distance involved. Nurses play a crucial role in preparing the patient for transport: they ensure that the patient is stable before departure, that all necessary equipment is available (oxygen, infusions, respiratory assistance devices), and that the patient is comfortable. They work closely with the medical transport teams, who take over from them to monitor the patient during the transfer. Effective communication is essential to ensure that the transport team has all the information on the patient's condition, current treatments and specific instructions to be followed during the journey.

Psychological preparation of the patient is another important aspect of transfers, whether inter-departmental or inter-hospital. Patients may feel anxious about a transfer, particularly if their state of health is critical, or if the transfer involves moving away from their loved ones. As the patient's first point of contact, nursing assistants play an essential role in this human dimension. They can reassure patients by explaining the reasons for the transfer, answering their questions and providing emotional support. They can also ensure that the patient's loved ones are informed of the transfer and the steps to be taken to maintain contact with him/her.

Managing emergencies during transfer is a situation that nursing assistants need to anticipate. If a patient's condition deteriorates, they need to be able to react quickly by communicating with the medical teams concerned, whether for an internal or inter-hospital transfer. In some cases, immediate care may be required, and caregivers must be prepared to assist nurses or doctors in emergency procedures, such as administering medication or adjusting medical devices. Their training and responsiveness are therefore essential to ensure patient safety.

Post-transfer follow-up is also crucial. Once the patient has been transferred to the new department or hospital, care assistants must ensure that all the necessary information has been passed on correctly, and that continuity of care is ensured without disruption. Teams in the receiving department need to be fully informed of the specifics of the patient's case and current clinical condition, so that care can be adapted immediately and effectively.

  ○ Specific cases: Pediatrics in cardiology, care of the elderly

Cardiac care in pediatrics and in the elderly represents two very different worlds, each with its own specific needs and challenges. Both populations require a distinct approach, both medically and relationally. In pediatrics, the challenge is to meet the needs of vulnerable children, often with congenital heart defects, while reassuring and involving their parents. In geriatrics, the challenge is to care for elderly people, often frail and with co-morbidities, in a context of aging and functional decline. In both cases, the approach to cardiology care must be comprehensive, empathetic and adapted to the particularities of each age group.

Pediatrics in cardiology: Caring for our youngest patients

Pediatric cardiology differs from adult cardiology in the nature of the pathologies treated, which are often congenital malformations of the heart or cardiac anomalies that appear from birth. Children suffering from such pathologies have to cope with complex surgical procedures, rigorous medical follow-up and, sometimes, treatment extending over several years. Caring for these young patients requires specific expertise and great sensitivity in the way we interact with them and their families.

The relationship with the child is a key element in pediatrics. Unlike adults, children often do not have a clear understanding of their illness, and can be frightened by the hospital, care or pain. Nurses, at the heart of day-to-day care, need to establish a relationship of trust with these young patients. This requires reassuring gestures, words adapted to their level of understanding, and the creation of a calm, reassuring environment. Playing with children, answering their questions in a straightforward manner, and ensuring that they feel supported at every stage of their treatment are fundamental aspects of this care.

Parental involvement is also essential. Parents of a child hospitalized for heart disease face a psychologically difficult ordeal, marked by worry and anxiety. Nurses play a mediating role between the medical team and the family, explaining the course of care and answering parents' questions with patience and empathy. They must also encourage parents' participation in day-to-day care, whenever possible, so that the child feels cared for and the parents retain a sense of control and involvement in the healing process. Parents' psychological support is just as crucial as that of the child, as their emotional well-being directly affects the child's ability to feel secure.

Postoperative care after cardiac surgery is also a critical time in pediatric care. Children require close monitoring of their vital signs and pain management, as well as rigorous follow-up of the healing process. Nurses play a fundamental role in this phase, ensuring the child's comfort, monitoring for signs of infection or complications, and collaborating with medical teams to adjust treatments as clinical conditions evolve. Wound hygiene, gentle mobilization and pain management are an integral part of the care provided, with particular attention paid to the tolerance of treatments and the gradual resumption of activities.

Therapeutic education also plays an important role in the care of children with chronic heart disease. Children must gradually learn to understand their illness, respect certain rules of life and take part in their treatment. Nurses, in collaboration with nurses and doctors, take part in this education by explaining treatments, precautions to be taken and limitations on physical exertion in a playful and appropriate way. Support in this education helps prepare the child to grow up with the disease, while leading as normal a life as possible.

Caring for the elderly: Respecting frailty

In cardiology care for the elderly, the challenge is often to manage patients with multiple pathologies, in addition to their heart problems. Heart failure, rhythm disorders or coronary heart disease are common in the elderly, often in conjunction with conditions such as diabetes, hypertension or kidney disease. Aging accentuates the fragility of the cardiovascular system, and care must be adapted to this vulnerability.

Comprehensive care of the elderly involves managing not only their heart disease, but also their co-morbidities and functional needs. Elderly people hospitalized in cardiology may have difficulty mobilizing, feeding or hydrating themselves. Caregivers are at the heart of their day-to-day work, providing hygiene, nutrition and ensuring that patients maintain adequate hydration, while monitoring for signs of cardiac decompensation or electrolyte imbalance. They must also pay particular attention to pressure sore prevention in these often bedridden patients, by carrying out regular position changes and using adapted prevention devices.

Managing polymedication is another fundamental aspect of caring for the elderly. These patients often take several medications to treat their various conditions, and the risk of drug interactions is high. Caregivers need to be particularly vigilant when administering medication, monitoring for possible side effects and reporting any suspicious symptoms to the medical team. The elderly are often more sensitive to the adverse effects of treatments, and it is essential to ensure that drug tolerance is properly assessed on a daily basis.

Rehabilitation after a cardiac event in the elderly is a delicate but crucial stage. These patients require specially adapted care if they are to regain an acceptable level of functional autonomy. Caregivers play an essential role in supporting this rehabilitation, by encouraging gentle mobilization, helping patients to perform simple gestures and participating in re-education exercises. The aim is to avoid further loss of autonomy and prevent complications associated with prolonged bed rest, such as lung infections or thrombosis.

Communicating with the elderly, often psychologically weakened by their illness and sometimes socially isolated, requires a great deal of empathy. Some patients may be confused, or suffer from cognitive disorders linked to their age or state of health, making communication difficult. Caregivers need to be patient, use clear and appropriate language, and ensure that patients understand the care they are receiving. Respect for the patient's dignity and individuality is crucial in this relationship: every gesture must be explained, and the patient's autonomy preserved as far as possible.

Emotional support is particularly important when caring for the elderly. Many of them, faced with chronic illness, increasing physical limitations and loss of autonomy, may experience anxiety or depression. Caregivers, through their daily proximity to these patients, play a key role in identifying these emotional states and providing psychological support. A smile, a conversation, a moment's listening can make a significant difference to these patients, bringing them comfort at a time of fragility.

Chapter 8

The Legal and Ethical Aspects of Working in Cardiology

The caregiver's legal responsibilities

○ Legal framework for the nursing profession
The legal framework for the nursing profession is a set of rules and standards that define the rights, duties and responsibilities of this essential healthcare profession. It is a framework governing not only training, professional practice and ethics, but also the protection of patients and professionals. Caregivers play a fundamental role in the healthcare system, working in close proximity to patients, providing essential support tasks for nursing and medical care, and looking after their day-to-day well-being. However, the profession is governed by a strict legal framework to guarantee the safety of care, the quality of practices, and the protection of patients' rights.

Training and legal recognition of the profession

The path to becoming a nursing auxiliary is governed by precise standards. The Diplôme d'Etat d'Aide-soignant (DEAS) is the certification that enables you to legally practice this profession in France. This diploma is obtained following specific training at accredited training institutes, such as the Instituts de Formation d'Aides-Soignants (IFAS). Training lasts 10 to 12 months, and includes theoretical and practical instruction, as well as internships in hospitals or care facilities.

Training covers areas such as hygiene and comfort care, patient communication, infection management, care of vulnerable people, and first aid. The legislative framework requires that training be validated by the award of a state diploma, a sine qua non condition for practicing the profession. This guarantees that care assistants are trained to a precise set of skills, enabling them to intervene in a wide variety of situations, whether in hospitals, retirement homes or home care.

The caregiver's field of expertise

The nursing auxiliary's field of competence is defined by regulatory texts, in particular the French **Public Health Code**. The nursing auxiliary works under the responsibility of a nurse, according to strict ethical rules. They are responsible for providing basic care and comfort, such as helping patients with washing, dressing and feeding, monitoring their general condition, and assisting them with activities of daily living. The nursing auxiliary cannot diagnose or administer medical treatments, as these acts fall within the exclusive competence of doctors and nurses.

However, the caregiver may need to work closely with the nurse for certain interventions, such as taking vital vitals (temperature, blood pressure, respiratory rate), helping to position the patient, or monitoring clinical signs that may indicate a worsening state of health. If necessary, the caregiver must be able to alert the nurse or doctor for more specific care. The legal framework requires that these tasks be carried out in compliance with current care protocols and within the limits of the caregiver's field of competence.

The caregiver's professional liability

As a healthcare professional, the caregiver is subject to legal, ethical and deontological obligations. They must respect the fundamental principles governing the caregiver-patient relationship, notably respect for human dignity, confidentiality of medical information, and patients' right to autonomy and to make informed decisions about their own health.

Professional secrecy is one of the cardinal principles of the profession. Like other healthcare professionals, orderlies are bound by medical secrecy, which prohibits the disclosure of personal and medical information relating to patients. This obligation, governed by the French Penal Code and the French Public Health Code, applies to everything the orderly sees, hears or learns in the course of his duties. Violation of this secrecy can result in disciplinary, civil and criminal sanctions, ranging from suspension of the right to practice to fines and prison sentences. Respect for professional secrecy is essential to ensure patient confidence in the healthcare system.

The civil and criminal liability of orderlies is also governed by law. In the event of fault or negligence in the performance of their duties, orderlies can be held liable for damage caused to patients. This may involve errors in the care provided, omissions in supervision, or a failure to ensure patient safety. For example, if a caregiver fails to comply with a care protocol, resulting in a nosocomial infection in a patient, he or she may be held liable. The legal framework therefore requires caregivers to respect the rules of the art and the protocols in force to minimize the risk of harm.

When it comes to **patient rights**, caregivers must also respect essential legal principles. Every patient has the right to quality care, respect and dignity. Caregivers must ensure that patients are clearly informed about the care they are to receive, and that they are able to give informed consent. This respect for patient autonomy is in line with the law on patients' rights and the quality of the healthcare system, known as the Kouchner law (2002). Thus, the caregiver must always ensure that the care he or she provides respects the patient's wishes, unless the patient's state of health prevents such dialogue.

Protection for orderlies

The legal framework for the nursing profession is not limited to professional obligations: it also includes protective measures for the caregivers themselves. Caregivers, who are exposed to physical, emotional and health risks in the course of their duties, benefit from specific protections, particularly in terms of occupational health.

Occupational risks, such as musculoskeletal disorders, nosocomial infections and stress in the workplace, are covered by occupational health legislation. Healthcare establishments are required to implement preventive measures to limit these risks, such as ergonomic training to reduce injuries when mobilizing patients, access to personal protective equipment (PPE), and strict hygiene protocols to prevent contamination.

In addition, care assistants benefit from a **right of withdrawal** in the event of serious and imminent danger to their health or safety. This enables them to suspend their activities without being penalized if working conditions present a significant risk, provided this right is exercised within the framework defined by law. Like all healthcare professionals, orderlies can also call on psychological support systems in the event of trauma linked to serious events occurring in the course of their work, particularly in intensive care or emergency units.

Changes in the legal framework

Finally, the legal framework for the nursing profession is constantly evolving to adapt to the realities of practice and the new challenges facing the healthcare system. Recent reforms aim to broaden the skills of nursing assistants, particularly in the context of managing dependency linked to an ageing population and homecare. Legislation is also tending to strengthen recognition of this profession, both in terms of skills and working conditions, with regular discussions on remuneration, skills enhancement and career development opportunities.

- ○ Notions of task delegation and shared responsibility

The notion of task delegation and shared responsibility lies at the heart of the organization of care in healthcare establishments. It reflects the need for close collaboration between different healthcare professionals, while guaranteeing patient safety and quality of care. In a hospital or homecare environment, each player - doctor, nurse, care assistant - has a well-defined role, but delegation enables certain tasks to be shared out to improve the efficiency of care, while respecting each professional's field of competence. Delegation of tasks therefore implies a strict framework, in which responsibilities are shared, but not diluted, between the different team members.

What is task delegation?

Delegation of tasks involves one healthcare professional entrusting another, under certain conditions, with acts that initially fall within his or her own remit. In the majority of cases, this occurs between a nurse and an orderly, since the orderly acts under the nurse's responsibility, but it can also occur in teams where a doctor delegates certain tasks to a nurse, or between a nursing manager and more junior caregivers. Delegation is governed by the French **Public Health Code**, which defines the conditions under which it can occur.

Delegation is not a simple allocation of tasks: it is the result of a carefully considered and supervised decision. Indeed, **delegation is only possible when the act in question corresponds to skills that the delegate can master**, according to his or her training and field of activity. Furthermore, delegation must always be in the patient's interest, and must in no way compromise the quality or safety of care. The delegator, often the nurse in the case of orderlies, remains responsible for the supervision and quality of the act performed. Delegation of tasks therefore relies on mutual trust, shared skills and fluid communication between the different professionals.

Acts that can be delegated

As part of their role in supporting nursing care, orderlies can be delegated several types of tasks. These tasks mainly concern

basic care and comfort, such as grooming, dressing, meal distribution, and accompanying patients in their daily activities. But as part of the delegation, they may also be entrusted with more technical acts, such as **taking vital signs** (blood pressure, temperature, respiratory rate), **monitoring infusions,** or helping to manage medical devices (probes, drains, catheters).

However, certain procedures **cannot be delegated**. For example, procedures requiring diagnosis, clinical interpretation or highly specific skills are reserved for doctors or nurses. Placing an infusion, administering injectable medication, or assessing pain at a complex level are all examples of acts that cannot be delegated to a caregiver. This ensures that medical procedures requiring advanced clinical expertise are carried out only by the most qualified professionals, thereby ensuring patient safety.

Delegation conditions

For delegation to be legitimate and effective, several conditions must be met. **The first condition is the assessment of the delegatee's competence**. Nurses who delegate a task to a caregiver must ensure that the latter has the knowledge and practice required to perform the act safely. This may include specific training or practical assessment, particularly in the case of technical procedures such as taking vital signs or monitoring a patient wearing a particular medical device.

The second condition is supervision of the delegator. The delegating professional remains responsible for the procedure he or she entrusts to another. In this context, he or she must ensure that the procedure is carried out correctly, and that there are no complications for the patient. This supervision can take different forms: it can be direct, with real-time monitoring of the procedure, or indirect, with a posteriori control of the quality of care. The nurse, for example, must check the vital signs measured by the orderly, and ensure that these are correctly recorded in the medical record.

The third condition is patient information. The delegation of a procedure must always respect the patient and his or her rights. The patient must be informed of the identity of the caregiver carrying out the care, and of each person's responsibilities. This is part of respecting patients' autonomy and their right to be cared for by competent professionals.

Shared responsibility

Under delegation, **responsibility is shared between the delegator and the delegatee**, but is clearly defined. The delegator, who is generally a nurse or health executive, remains responsible for the overall act, even if he or she did not perform the act directly. He or she is responsible for ensuring that the procedure is carried out correctly, that the delegate's skills are appropriate, and that the patient is safe. Thus, if a problem arises as a result of delegation, the delegator can be held responsible for poor assessment of skills or lack of supervision.

The delegate, **for** his part, is **responsible for the act he performs**. If he accepts a delegation, he must ensure that he respects good practice and follows the protocols in force. If the caregiver accepts a task for which he or she does not feel competent, or performs the act incorrectly by neglecting procedures, his or her individual responsibility may be engaged. It is therefore crucial that the delegate feels confident and trained to accept delegation.

This **shared responsibility** does not mean that roles become confused. Each professional remains within his or her own field of competence, and delegation should enable care to flow more smoothly without compromising quality. Delegation is not a transfer of responsibility, but rather a sharing of care, where each individual remains responsible for his or her own part of the work.

Delegating tasks within a multidisciplinary framework

In a multi-disciplinary team, delegating tasks makes perfect sense. It enables the **workload** to be **better distributed** between team members, and optimizes the time and skills of each member. For example, a nurse can delegate certain monitoring or comfort care tasks to an orderly, allowing him or her to concentrate on more technical and complex medical procedures. The result is a better quality of care, with each professional working within the scope of his or her skills.

In addition, task delegation strengthens **trust and collaboration within teams**. It implies mutual respect for each other's skills and recognition of the importance of different roles in overall patient care. Delegating shows recognition of each other's skills and a shared commitment to quality care.

　　　　　◦　　The limits of caregiver intervention
The nursing auxiliary's role is essential to the smooth running of the healthcare system, but it is clearly defined by legal, ethical and practical boundaries. Although caregivers play a key role in accompanying patients and providing basic care, they can only intervene within a framework strictly defined by law and under the responsibility of the nurse or doctor. These limits are there to guarantee patient safety, avoid medical errors and ensure that each healthcare professional intervenes according to his or her skills and level of training. By understanding and respecting these limits, the nursing auxiliary contributes to the quality of care, while ensuring the consistency and safety of treatment.

Legal framework and jurisdiction

One of the foundations on which the limits of the nursing auxiliary's interventions are based is the **legal framework** and its **field of competence**, clearly defined by the French **Public Health**

Code. This framework specifies the acts that caregivers are authorized to perform, and those that fall within the exclusive competence of other healthcare professionals, notably doctors and nurses.

The caregiver's tasks mainly concern **hygiene and comfort care**, such as helping with washing, dressing and eating, and mobilizing patients to prevent bedsores or facilitate movement. Although essential, this care involves neither medical diagnosis nor complex therapeutic treatment.

The nursing auxiliary is also authorized to carry out certain **simple monitoring tasks**, such as taking temperatures, measuring blood pressure or monitoring the patient's general condition (change in skin color, agitation, signs of pain). However, such monitoring must be reported to the nurse or physician, who is responsible for interpreting the data and making clinical decisions.

Medical procedures: an insurmountable limit

The nursing auxiliary **cannot** diagnose, prescribe medication or perform medical procedures requiring clinical expertise. For example, **setting up an infusion**, administering intravenous medication, or intubating a patient in respiratory distress fall exclusively within the remit of a nurse or doctor. Similarly, the clinical assessment of signs of serious deterioration, such as acute pulmonary edema or myocardial infarction, cannot be carried out by the orderly.

These limits are justified by the need to protect patients' health and ensure that the most complex procedures are carried out by professionals with in-depth training and the ability to react to critical situations. **Legal liability** in the event of negligence or error during a medical procedure is high, and if the orderly exceeds his or her competence, he or she may be held responsible for any harm caused to the patient.

Delegation under supervision

Although certain actions can be delegated to a caregiver by a nurse or doctor, this is only done if they fall within the **caregiver's field of competence**. For example, a nurse may ask an orderly to monitor a patient's condition after surgery, check his or her temperature or change his or her dressings. However, the nurse remains responsible for supervising these acts and assessing the patient's condition. The orderly cannot make clinical decisions on the basis of his or her observations, but must report any anomalies or changes in condition to the professionals in charge.

In addition, it is important to remember that **the caregiver can refuse a task if it exceeds his or her competence**, or if he or she feels that he or she has not received sufficient training to carry it out safely. This ability to refuse a task deemed inappropriate or dangerous is crucial to avoid errors and protect both the patient and the caregiver himself/herself from possible legal consequences.

Emergency management

In the course of their work, carers may be confronted with emergency situations such as cardiac arrest, epileptic seizures or haemorrhage. In such circumstances, it is essential to understand that the caregiver cannot **intervene directly with specialized medical care**, but can provide first aid while waiting for the medical team to intervene.

For example, in the event of cardiac arrest, the caregiver can initiate first aid measures such as cardiopulmonary resuscitation (CPR) and the use of an automated external defibrillator (AED) if the equipment is available. However, administering medication or intubating a patient are medical procedures reserved for nurses or doctors.

In the event of **respiratory distress**, the caregiver can help reposition the patient, administer oxygen under the supervision of a nurse, but cannot alone decide on the administration of specific treatment or the use of invasive techniques.

These emergency situations underline another essential limitation of caregivers' interventions: although they are often on the front line in identifying problems, **they cannot intervene beyond their training**, but must quickly alert qualified professionals to manage the situation optimally.

Relational and ethical aspects

The limits of the nursing auxiliary's interventions concern not only technical acts, but also **relational aspects**. In their relations with patients, caregivers must respect their privacy, dignity and autonomy. They cannot, for example, force a patient to accept a treatment, or make decisions on behalf of the patient or his or her family. All steps taken must respect the patient's rights, including the right to refuse care.

Professional secrecy is another important limitation. Caregivers are bound by absolute medical secrecy, and may under no circumstances divulge information concerning a patient's state of health, except to professionals directly involved in the care. Violation of this rule may result in criminal and disciplinary sanctions. Furthermore, even in situations where relatives request information, the caregiver may not divulge details of the patient's health without the patient's explicit consent or the doctors' authorization.

Evolving skills and new challenges

Although the scope of a nursing auxiliary's work is clearly defined, it is important to emphasize that the **skills of these professionals evolve** over time. As the population ages and care becomes increasingly complex, caregivers are increasingly called upon to manage complex situations, particularly in the context of home care or nursing homes.

For example, there is currently a debate on extending the skills of nursing assistants, notably through continuing training and specific certifications that would enable them to carry out additional technical acts under the supervision of nurses, particularly in the fields of **gerontology** or **palliative care**. However, any extension of these competencies will always have to take place within a rigorous legislative framework, ensuring that patient safety remains the top priority.

Ethical care in cardiology

     ◦   Common ethical dilemmas in cardiology: therapeutic overkill, refusal of care, etc.

Ethical dilemmas in cardiology are complex situations that place fundamental principles of care in tension, such as respect for life, dignity, patient autonomy and medical responsibility. These dilemmas frequently arise in the context of serious, chronic pathologies, where therapeutic decisions can have profound physical and psychological consequences for patients and their families. Among the most sensitive issues are those of therapeutic overkill, refusal of care, end-of-life care and advance directives. These situations raise questions about the limits of medical treatment and the place of patients' wishes in decision-making.

Therapeutic overkill: Where do we draw the line?

Therapeutic obstinacy, sometimes referred to as unreasonable obstinacy, is one of the main ethical issues that arise in cardiology, especially in the case of patients at the end of life or suffering from severely debilitating chronic illnesses. Therapeutic overkill refers to the continuation or initiation of medical treatments deemed disproportionate to the patient's condition, with little or no hope of improvement or recovery, while prolonging unnecessary suffering.

In cardiology, this situation often arises in the context of elderly patients with end-stage heart failure or severe cardiac pathologies. These patients may be subjected to heavy treatments, such as invasive surgery, cardiac assistance devices, or repeated hospitalizations in intensive care, without any real improvement in their quality of life. The ethical question then arises: how far should we go to maintain life, and at what point should we recognize that continued care becomes a form of therapeutic obstinacy, prolonging biological life to the detriment of the patient's overall well-being?

For healthcare professionals, the dividing line between legitimate treatment and therapeutic obstinacy is often blurred. In France, the **Leonetti-Claeys law** specifies that care must not be continued when it is unreasonable and when it offers no benefit in terms of quality of life for the patient. It also introduces the right to deep and continuous sedation at the end of life to avoid unnecessary suffering. However, the application of these principles remains difficult in daily practice. Health-care teams have to take into account the expectations of families, who may find it difficult to accept that the end of life is imminent, while respecting the wishes of patients themselves. Caregivers, who maintain a close relationship with patients, can sometimes find themselves witnessing these tensions and questioning the appropriateness of the care administered.

Refusal of care: Respecting patient autonomy

Refusal of care is another major ethical dilemma in cardiology. It arises when a patient, informed of his or her state of health and the therapeutic options available, chooses not to follow the proposed course of treatment, even though this refusal may have serious or even fatal consequences. In cardiology, this can take the form of refusing heart surgery or drug treatment for heart failure, or rejecting the hospitalization required to stabilize the patient's condition.

The **patient's right to autonomy** is a fundamental principle of medical ethics and is enshrined in law. Every patient has the right to make decisions concerning his or her own body and care, even if these decisions run counter to the recommendations of healthcare professionals. However, this autonomy must be informed: doctors and nurses have a duty to inform patients clearly and fully of the risks involved in refusing care. If the patient understands what is at stake but persists in his or her choice, the caregiver is faced with a moral dilemma: respecting the patient's decision while knowing that it may lead to a rapid deterioration in his or her condition, or even death.

This dilemma can be even more complex when the patient has cognitive impairments or impaired judgment. For example, an elderly patient suffering from dementia may refuse essential care without fully understanding the consequences of his or her decision. In such cases, the role of caregivers and family becomes crucial, but the question of how far to respect the patient's wishes remains open.

For caregivers, who are often in direct and prolonged contact with patients, refusal of care can be difficult to manage. Their close relationship with the patient can make them feel powerless in the face of refusal, especially if the patient expresses pain or discomfort while rejecting the help offered. The caregiver's role in these situations is to support the patient, respecting his or her choices, while relaying essential information to the medical team so that dialogue with the patient can remain open.

Care at the end of life: Relief without prolongation

End-of-life cardiology is another area where many ethical dilemmas arise. For patients with advanced heart disease, such as refractory heart failure or complex coronary pathologies, the question often arises as to when to stop curative treatments and concentrate solely on palliative care. Palliative care aims to relieve pain and improve quality of life, without artificially prolonging life.

The transition to palliative care can be difficult to accept for families, who may feel that the decision has been abandoned. However, it is often the best way to preserve the patient's dignity and avoid over-treatment. Palliative care makes it possible to manage symptoms such as chest pain, dyspnea or anxiety without resorting to invasive treatments that would only prolong suffering.

Caregivers play a crucial role in this phase, as they are often the ones who accompany the patient in his last moments of life. They are responsible for keeping the patient comfortable, ensuring hydration, pain management and general well-being. They are also there to offer emotional and psychological support to both patient and family, helping them through this difficult period. The ethical dilemma for caregivers can arise when they have to accept that, despite their best efforts, the patient's death is inevitable, and that it is sometimes preferable to prioritize quality at the end of life rather than prolonging it at all costs.

Advance directives and shared decision-making

Advance directives are a way for patients to express their wishes regarding the end of their lives, particularly in the event of loss of consciousness or inability to communicate. In cardiology, these directives enable patients to specify in advance whether or not they wish to receive certain treatments, such as cardiopulmonary resuscitation, intubation or the use of cardiac assistance devices.

When advance directives are clear and present in the medical record, they can help resolve certain ethical dilemmas by sparing caregivers and families from having to make difficult decisions without knowing the patient's wishes. However, in many cases, these directives are not written down or do not cover all possible situations. This leaves medical teams and families in a state of uncertainty, forcing them to make decisions in real time, often under emotionally-charged conditions.

The **principle of shared decision-making** aims to involve patients, when they are still able to do so, in discussions about their care. The aim is to strike a balance between medical recommendations and the patient's wishes, respecting both his or her autonomy and the principle of beneficence, which urges caregivers to act for the patient's own good. This approach often helps to clarify priorities: relieving suffering, maintaining a certain quality of life, or, in some cases, accepting that death is part of the natural process.

- ∘ The caregiver-patient relationship: Respect, dignity and autonomy

The relationship between caregiver and patient is at the heart of nursing practice, and is based on essential values such as respect, dignity and the promotion of autonomy. This relationship is particularly unique in that it involves daily proximity to the patient, a direct and prolonged contact that goes far beyond the simple provision of technical care. The caregiver is often the one who accompanies patients in the most intimate daily gestures, while ensuring their comfort, well-being and dignity. In this relationship, respect for the individual, attention to their needs, and the desire to preserve their autonomy are the fundamental principles that guide the caregiver's actions.

Respect at the heart of the relationship

Respect is the essential foundation of any caregiver-patient relationship. It means treating each patient as an individual, with his or her own needs, desires, beliefs and life stories. For the caregiver, this means paying particular attention to the way he or she interacts with the patient, respecting his or her preferences and taking account of his or her emotions and frailties. Respect is shown through simple but essential gestures: knocking before entering the room, using an appropriate tone of voice, addressing the patient by name, and above all, listening to his or her needs without judgment.

In day-to-day practice, this respect is also reflected in the caregiver's attitude to acts of care. For example, when helping a patient to wash or dress, the caregiver must be careful to respect the patient's privacy, ensuring the necessary discretion. It's important to ensure that the patient doesn't feel infantilized or reduced to his or her medical needs. This respectful approach helps to create a climate of trust and security, where the patient feels valued as a person.

Respect also includes respecting the patient's **rhythm**. Each individual his has or her own pace, whether it's getting up, eating or performing personal care. The caregiver, although often working in a time-constrained environment, must be able to adapt to this rhythm, taking the time needed to carry out care in a calm and reassuring manner. By respecting these aspects, the caregiver shows that he or she considers the patient as a whole, and not just as a patient to be treated.

Dignity: preserving the patient's humanity

Maintaining the patient's dignity is another fundamental pillar of the caregiver-patient relationship. Human dignity is an inalienable right, and must never be compromised, even in situations where the patient is highly dependent or vulnerable. In the hospital or care facility environment, patients are often confronted with loss of control over their bodies, their health, and sometimes even their daily lives. This can lead to a loss of self-esteem and great emotional fragility.

In this context, the caregiver has a crucial role to play in helping to maintain the patient's dignity. This begins with **attention to privacy**. When intimate care is to be provided, the caregiver ensures that the patient is not exposed unnecessarily, uses screens or sheets to preserve modesty, and explains each gesture before carrying it out, so that the patient understands what is going to happen and does not feel objectified. It is also essential that the caregiver takes into account the patient's feelings and respects his or her limits: if a patient expresses discomfort during a treatment, the treatment must be adapted to avoid any humiliation.

Patient dignity also means **respecting the patient's voice** and decisions. Even in highly dependent situations, the patient must be consulted and informed of what is happening, and his or her voice must be heard. This means that the caregiver must explain the care he or she is providing and ensure that the patient consents to it. For example, in the case of toileting, the patient must be able to choose whether he or she wants to wash now or later, or how he or she prefers to be helped. This respect for patients' dignity enables them to retain a degree of control and autonomy over their own lives, even in the event of illness.

Autonomy: encouragement and support

One of the fundamental aims of the caregiver-patient relationship is to **promote and maintain the patient's autonomy**, wherever possible. Autonomy is the ability of each individual to make informed choices and carry out the acts of daily life independently. Illness, aging or hospitalization can limit this autonomy, but the caregiver plays an important role in helping the patient maintain, or even regain, a certain degree of independence.

Promoting autonomy means first and foremost encouraging patients to do what they are capable of doing on their own, even if this may take time or require supervision. For example, a patient who has just undergone an operation may be able to wash himself partially on his own, or move around with limited assistance. In such cases, the caregiver must encourage the patient to carry out these tasks on his or her own, while remaining at the patient's side to help out if necessary. This approach not only prevents further loss of autonomy, but also restores the patient's confidence in his or her own abilities.

In some cases, illness or age can impose severe limitations on autonomy. In this context, it is essential that the caregiver adapts his or her care to the patient's remaining capacities, without ever imposing excessive assistance that could disempower the patient. **Teamwork** with physiotherapists or occupational therapists is crucial here, to promote functional rehabilitation and the patient's gradual autonomy.

Autonomy also concerns the patient's ability to participate actively in his or her own care and medical decisions. The caregiver, in liaison with the medical team, must ensure that the patient is clearly and appropriately informed about his or her state of health and the care he or she is receiving. Patients must be encouraged to ask questions, express their preferences and participate in the development of their care plan. In doing so, the caregiver respects the patient's dignity by enabling them to play an active role in their care, while reinforcing their sense of autonomy and control.

○ Cases of conscience: Practical examples and ethical solutions

Cases of conscience in the medical environment, and more specifically in the day-to-day work of care assistants, arise when decisions have to be made in the face of situations that conflict with different ethical principles. These situations may concern respect for the patient's wishes, the dilemma between prolonging life at all costs or relieving suffering, or how to reconcile professional constraints with the humanity required for care. Each case of conscience requires profound ethical reflection, where the ideal solution is not always obvious. Here are a few practical examples that illustrate these dilemmas and the ethical solutions envisaged to overcome them.

Conscientious case 1: The patient refuses treatment

A classic example of a case of conscience concerns a patient's refusal of care. Let's imagine an elderly patient suffering from heart failure, who systematically refuses the grooming and daily care offered by the nursing team. He says he doesn't want to be disturbed, but his refusal of care could lead to medical complications, such as skin infections or bedsores. For the caregiver, the situation becomes delicate: should he respect the patient's choice, at the risk of endangering his health, or should he insist on providing care despite this refusal?

Ethical solution: The first step in resolving this dilemma is to respect the patient's right to autonomy, which is a fundamental principle. Refusal of care must be listened to, but this does not mean that caregivers should give up. The solution is to enter into a dialogue with the patient to understand the underlying reasons for refusal. Is he embarrassed by the loss of intimacy that care represents? Is he afraid of pain or dependency? By identifying the causes of the refusal, the caregiver can adapt his or her approach, suggest alternatives (later care, light care, etc.) and reassure the patient about his or her fears.

If, despite everything, the patient continues to refuse care, it is essential to remember that, except in cases of serious endangerment, the patient's choice must be respected. However, the situation must be reported to the medical team for an overall assessment, and follow-up must be maintained to avoid the serious consequences of prolonged refusal.

Case study 2: Pain at the end of life

Another frequently encountered case of conscience concerns the management of pain in a patient at the end of life. Let's imagine a palliative care patient suffering from terminal cancer, who expresses great physical suffering and asks caregivers to increase the dose of morphine to relieve her pain. However, increasing analgesic doses could lead to deep sedation, or even hasten the patient's death. The caregiver, who accompanies this patient on a daily basis, is faced with a dilemma: to respect the patient's request for relief, or to fear indirectly contributing to the end of her life.

Ethical solution: In this type of situation, the ethical principle of **beneficence**, which implies alleviating the patient's suffering, comes into conflict with the principle of **non-maleficence**, which is to do no harm. The solution lies in an approach centered on the patient's wishes and the law on palliative care. In France, the Leonetti-Claeys law authorizes deep and continuous sedation at the end of life in cases where the patient's suffering is refractory to standard treatments.

The caregiver, in consultation with the medical team, must ensure that the patient is fully informed of the consequences of increasing morphine doses, and that this decision is taken in an informed manner. It is also essential to involve the family in this discussion, while respecting the patient's wishes. The most important thing is to put the patient's quality of life and dignity first. In this context, increasing doses to relieve suffering should not be perceived as a desire to hasten death, but as an act of compassion and respect for the patient's dignity.

Case study 3: Prolonging life or accepting the end

Another frequent case of conscience in cardiology is that of frail, elderly patients who, after several hospitalizations and operations, find themselves in a situation of extreme dependence and physical exhaustion. Imagine a patient suffering from advanced heart failure, who has already undergone several major surgical procedures, and who expresses his exhaustion in the face of intensive care and invasive treatments. The family, on the other hand, insists on continuing care, hoping for improvement despite a very bleak prognosis. The patient, tired and aware of his condition, simply wants us to stop the active treatments and let him go with dignity. The caregiver, who assists this patient on a daily basis, feels the patient's psychological suffering, but finds himself in a dilemma when faced with contradictory demands between the patient's wishes and the pressure of the family.

Ethical solution: This case illustrates the conflict between **respecting the patient's wishes** and the difficulty for loved ones of letting a loved one go. The caregiver, in this context, must respect the patient's wishes, as the law grants every individual the right to refuse treatment, including prolonged resuscitation. The caregiver's role here is to act as a benevolent mediator, helping to open a dialogue between the patient, the nursing team and the family. He or she can encourage a consultation with the referring physician to clarify the situation and explain that the priority must be the patient's quality of life, rather than over-zealous treatment.

In this situation, psychological support for the family is crucial to enable them to accept the patient's decision. The caregiver's empathetic attitude can help ease tensions and create a climate in which the patient's decision is heard and respected, while ensuring that the patient receives palliative care adapted to his or her situation.

Case study 4: Confidentiality in emergency situations

Let's imagine that a caregiver is looking after a young patient who has suffered a heart attack and is hospitalized in intensive care. During his daily care, the patient confides in the caregiver important personal information about his addiction problems, which may have contributed to his current condition. He asks the caregiver to keep this confidential. However, this information could be crucial for adjusting medical treatment and preventing possible complications. The caregiver is then faced with a dilemma: to respect professional secrecy and the confidentiality of the patient's confidences, or to share this information with the medical team to protect the patient's health.

Ethical solution: Professional secrecy is a fundamental principle in the doctor-patient relationship, and it is essential that patients are able to confide in us without fear that their personal information will be divulged. However, the **duty of beneficence** and patient safety may justify a partial waiver of this secrecy, provided this is in the patient's direct interest.

In this case, the caregiver can explain to the patient that this information could have an impact on his or her treatment, and that it would be beneficial to discuss it with the medical team. The caregiver should seek the patient's consent before sharing this information. If the patient categorically refuses, the caregiver can discreetly consult a member of the medical team, such as a doctor or psychologist, to assess the situation in greater depth, without betraying the patient's trust, but taking care to protect his or her health.

Medical error and incident management

◦   Recognizing and reporting medical errors

Recognizing and reporting medical errors is a crucial aspect of healthcare practice, and is particularly important in the healthcare sector, where patient safety must always be a priority. Medical errors can occur at various levels of the care process: drug administration, incorrect patient identification, documentation or communication errors, or failure to comply with safety protocols. Although error is part of the human condition, it can have serious consequences in the medical environment. Recognizing and reporting these errors is essential to improving practices, preventing their recurrence and, above all, protecting patients.

Types of medical errors

Medical errors can take many forms. They concern not only the actions of doctors, but also those of the entire healthcare team, including orderlies. Here are some common examples of medical errors:

1.   **Medication error**: An error in the prescribing, preparation or administration of a medication. This can include the

wrong dose, the wrong form of medication (tablet instead of solution), or administration to the wrong patient.

2. **Communication errors**: This category of errors relates to poorly transmitted information between members of the healthcare team, whether when passing instructions between teams, or when transmitting information to the patient. Poor communication can lead to errors in care or delays in necessary treatment.

3. **Procedural error**: This may involve poorly performed technical care (e.g. incorrectly inserted infusion), failure to comply with hygiene protocols, or omission of certain monitoring procedures that could prevent patient complications.

4. **Identification error**: This error occurs when care is administered to the wrong person, due to insufficient or incorrect patient identification.

Recognition of medical errors

Recognizing a medical error requires **constant vigilance** and keen observation. Because of their proximity to patients and their regular presence on nursing teams, orderlies are often on the front line when it comes to identifying errors, whether in administering care, managing records or observing the patient's clinical signs.

Clinical observation is a key tool for detecting certain errors. For example, if a patient shows signs of deterioration after receiving a drug treatment, it's possible that the drug was incorrectly dosed or administered by mistake. Similarly, a patient whose condition does not improve after technical care could signal that something has not been done correctly. In this context, caregivers need to pay close attention and alert immediately when they notice an anomaly.

Systematic auditing of practices is another way of preventing or recognizing errors. Before administering care or assisting a patient, it is essential to ensure that everything corresponds to medical prescriptions: check the patient's identity, the nature of the treatment to be administered, and make sure that the protocol in force is respected.

Finally, **confidence in** safety **procedures and tools**, such as double-checking (cross-checking of medications by two people) or the use of patient identification bracelets, is fundamental to minimizing the risk of errors.

Reporting medical errors

Once an error has been identified, it is essential to **report** it **promptly**. Although it may seem difficult or uncomfortable, reporting an error is an essential step in correcting it, limiting its consequences and preventing it from happening again.

1. **Inform the team immediately**: If the error is in progress or has just occurred, the priority is to stop it and immediately inform members of the healthcare team, including the nurse or doctor in charge. This enables corrective action to be taken, such as administering an antidote, adjusting a treatment or monitoring the patient more closely to prevent possible complications.

2. **Document the error**: Reporting an error also requires clear, precise documentation in the patient's file. It is essential to **record exactly what happened**, without trying to minimize or embellish the facts. This transparency enables other team members to understand the situation and adjust care accordingly.

3. **Completing an incident report** : Most healthcare facilities have set up systems for **reporting adverse events**. These reports enable errors to be reported anonymously or not, and the incident to be recorded as

part of a continuous improvement process. This report is essential, as it enables weaknesses in existing practices or protocols to be detected and remedied to prevent the error from recurring.

4. **Informing the patient**: Patients have the right to be informed when an error occurs in their care, especially if it has consequences for their health. Transparency is crucial to maintaining trust between patients and caregivers. Whenever possible, information should be conveyed by the doctor or a professional empowered to explain the medical implications of the error, but the caregiver can also play a role by offering empathetic support to the patient after the incident.

Barriers to error reporting

Reporting errors can sometimes come up against psychological or organizational obstacles. Fear of disciplinary sanctions, a poor professional image or a loss of confidence on the part of colleagues or superiors can dissuade a caregiver from reporting an error. Yet **the culture of patient safety is** based on the idea that acknowledging errors, rather than hiding them, is a lever for improvement, not a source of blame.

To overcome these obstacles, it is crucial to promote a **culture of transparency and non-blaming** within healthcare facilities. It is essential that every team member feels encouraged to report errors without fear of negative repercussions. Medical errors should be seen as opportunities for learning and future prevention, not as personal failures.

The positive consequences of error reporting

Reporting errors has positive effects on several levels. Firstly, **it protects the patient** by taking prompt corrective action. Secondly, it offers the healthcare team the opportunity to learn from the incident and improve practices to prevent the error from recurring.

At a broader level, **incident reports** enable hospitals and care facilities to identify trends and critical points in their procedures. For example, if several medication errors occur in the same department, this may indicate that prescribing or administration practices need to be re-evaluated. This helps to improve protocols and reinforce the training of care teams.

Last but not least, **transparency** towards patients and families reinforces trust in the healthcare system. Patients are often more understanding than we think, especially when they feel they are being cared for honestly and respectfully. A proactive approach to error management can even improve the doctor-patient relationship.

◦   How to respond to a critical incident

When a critical incident occurs in a care environment, the way to react quickly and effectively is crucial to patient safety and well-being. A critical incident can include situations such as cardiac arrest, a serious patient fall, haemorrhage, or any other emergency directly endangering a patient's life or health. Faced with these events, every second counts, and caregivers, including orderlies, need to know how to react in a coordinated and calm manner. It's not just a question of acting quickly, but also methodically, following established protocols to minimize risk and maximize the patient's chances of survival or stabilization.

Stay calm and assess the situation

When a critical incident occurs, the first reaction must be to **remain calm**. This may seem counter-intuitive in an emergency situation, but it's essential to avoid any panic that could interfere with an accurate assessment of the situation. As a caregiver, presence of mind is crucial to effective action. You need to quickly get an **overview of** the situation: what is the immediate problem? Is the patient conscious? Is he or she breathing? Are there any obvious signs of deterioration, such as bleeding, loss of consciousness or severe chest pain? This initial, rapid assessment enables you to decide what action to take without wasting time.

For example, if a patient shows symptoms of cardiac arrest (unconsciousness, lack of breathing, pulse not perceptible), it is essential to **react immediately** to initiate resuscitation. If, on the other hand, the incident involves a fall, you must first assess whether the patient is conscious and check for serious injuries before moving the person.

Alert the medical team

Rapid communication with the medical team is one of the first reflexes to adopt. After assessing the seriousness of the situation, the caregiver must immediately **alert the appropriate personnel**. Depending on the seriousness of the incident, this often involves contacting the referring nurse, a doctor or the internal emergency services. The message must be clear and concise, explaining the nature of the incident and the patient's condition.

For example, in the event of cardiac arrest, the caregiver must immediately report that a patient is in respiratory arrest and requires cardiopulmonary resuscitation (CPR). It is important to provide essential details, such as the time of the incident and the signs observed (absence of breathing, skin discoloration, etc.). This communication enables the medical team to react appropriately and provide the necessary care quickly.

Administer first aid measures

While the caregiver alerts the other team members, **first aid** must be initiated if it's within the caregiver's area of expertise. In the case of cardiac arrest, this means immediately starting **cardiopulmonary resuscitation (CPR)** while waiting for the medical team to arrive with a defibrillator. Caregivers are trained in this lifesaving technique, and knowing how to apply it in good time can save lives. It's essential to follow resuscitation protocols: chest compressions at a rapid rate (100 to 120 compressions per minute), interspersed with ventilations if possible.

In the event of a **serious fall** or incident involving physical trauma, the caregiver must ensure that the patient is not moved until his or her condition has been assessed by more qualified professionals, unless the situation presents an imminent danger (for example, a fall in a dangerous environment or a fire). If the patient is bleeding, the first step is to **compress the bleeding area** to prevent massive hemorrhage.

In each case, the **caregiver** must know his or her **limits of intervention**, and know when to stop an action that goes beyond his or her field of competence, to make way for the medical team.

Follow emergency protocols

Every healthcare facility has precise **emergency protocols** detailing the steps to be taken in the event of critical incidents. These protocols are designed to organize a coordinated and effective response to medical emergencies. As a member of the healthcare team, the orderly must be familiar with these procedures and apply them rigorously.

For example, in the event of a fire, an alarm must be triggered, staff must be mobilized to evacuate patients safely, and effective communication must be put in place to ensure that all teams are kept informed. Similarly, in the event of a serious medical incident, the protocol may involve calling in reinforcements, preparing resuscitation equipment or implementing increased surveillance measures while waiting for specialized services to intervene.

Working as part of a team and supporting other caregivers

When faced with a critical incident, **team spirit** is essential. The orderly must not only focus on the immediate actions he or she can take, but also be ready to assist other members of the medical team once they are on the scene. This may mean helping to prepare medical equipment, monitoring other patients while the team responds, or simply providing additional information about the incident.

Coordination of efforts is vital to ensure that appropriate care is given without delay. For example, in a resuscitation context, a team may divide tasks: while one member performs chest compressions, another may administer oxygen, while a third prepares the defibrillator or medication.

The caregiver must also provide **emotional support to the patient**, if he or she is conscious, or to the relatives present. In a crisis situation, a word of comfort or a soothing gesture can help calm a person in distress. In some cases, relatives may be disoriented and stricken-panic, and the caregiver must manage this human dimension by reassuring and informing.

Post-crisis management: Follow-up and documentation

Once the critical incident has been brought under control and the patient is under the care of the medical teams, the role of the caregiver doesn't stop there. Post-incident **follow-up** is crucial to ensure continuity of care and prevent possible complications. The caregiver must continue to observe the patient's condition, ensure that all comfort and monitoring measures are in place, and maintain a safe environment.

What's more, **documenting the incident** is a mandatory step. The caregiver must complete an incident report, detailing precisely what happened, how the situation was handled, and the actions taken. This documentation enables the care team to analyze the situation, understand the causes of the incident and, if necessary, improve protocols for the future.

Post-incident reflection is also important for staff. It is useful to debrief after a critical incident, to discuss what worked and what could be improved. This collective moment of reflection reinforces care practices and ensures better preparation for future emergencies.

    ○   Patient safety culture : Continuous improvement of practices

A culture of patient safety is a fundamental principle of any healthcare system. It aims to ensure that every patient receives quality care, in an environment where the risks of errors, incidents or complications are minimized as far as possible. This culture is based on a dynamic of continuous improvement of practices, which means not only preventing errors, but also identifying, analyzing and correcting system flaws to improve long-term safety. The culture of patient safety involves all players in the healthcare system, from doctors and orderlies to nurses and managers, and is based on the values of transparency, shared responsibility and vigilance.

The foundations of a patient safety culture

Patient safety is based on the idea that medical errors are not just individual faults, but can result from failures in the system, such as poor communication, inadequate protocols, or unfavorable working conditions. Consequently, the modern approach to patient safety focuses on improving processes and structures, rather than simply assigning individual responsibility. This systemic vision is essential to creating a safer care environment.

One of the central principles is the promotion of a **non-punitive culture**. This means that caregivers, including orderlies, must feel confident to report errors or incidents without fear of disciplinary repercussions. This approach promotes transparency, as errors can be analyzed constructively, enabling the whole team to learn from them. This framework encourages the active participation of all caregivers in identifying risks, proposing improvements and implementing new safety practices.

Open communication is another pillar of the patient safety culture. It implies that members of the healthcare team can freely exchange information on identified risks, errors made or procedures to be improved. Each member of the team must be able to share his or her observations, whether it's an orderly pointing out a potential risk, a nurse highlighting shortcomings in the transmission of instructions, or a doctor reviewing protocols. This open dialogue is essential to detect problems at an early stage and remedy them before they turn into incidents.

Daily vigilance: a key role for the caregiver

In day-to-day practice, the **vigilance** of caregivers is crucial to maintaining a high level of patient safety. As front-line workers, orderlies spend a great deal of time with patients, enabling them to detect early signs of complications or anomalies in the care provided. Their role goes beyond hygiene and comfort care: they are constant observers of changes in the patient's state of health.

For example, by regularly monitoring vital signs, caregivers can spot abnormal fluctuations in temperature or blood pressure and quickly alert the nursing team. Similarly, by paying close attention to the patient's reactions following the administration of a treatment, they can detect unexpected side effects or intolerance to the medication. This preventive vigilance is a key component of patient safety, as it helps prevent worsening health conditions before they become emergencies.

Continuous improvement of practices

Continuous improvement is based on a proactive approach to analyzing and optimizing care processes. This approach is often formalized through **internal audits, morbidity-mortality reviews** and **incident analysis**. Every incident or error is considered a learning opportunity, not a failure. For example, when a critical incident occurs, an in-depth analysis is carried out to understand the contributing factors (poor communication, inadequate protocol, work overload) and identify solutions to prevent the incident from recurring.

Caregivers play a key role in this process, sharing their experience and contributing ideas for improvement. Through their proximity to patients and their practical knowledge of care, they can provide important insights into the difficulties encountered on a daily basis. This may include suggestions on how to improve hygiene protocols, reduce medication errors, or facilitate communication between day and night teams. Their contribution is essential to adjusting practices to the realities on the ground.

Another important aspect of continuous improvement is **regular** staff **training**. As care practices evolve, care assistants, like the rest of the nursing staff, need to keep abreast of new protocols, updated care techniques, and regulatory developments in the field of safety. Attending regular training sessions enables caregivers to stay up to date and reinforce their ability to prevent errors. This includes training in **emergency procedures**, **medical device management** or the use of **new** patient **monitoring tools**.

The role of protocols in patient safety

Care protocols play a central role in the culture of patient safety. They are designed to standardize practices and ensure that every caregiver follows precise, validated steps to minimize the risk of error. These protocols cover a wide range of aspects, from the administration of medication to the management of nosocomial infections and the prevention of falls or bedsores.

In their day-to-day work, orderlies must adhere strictly to these protocols. For example, before administering care or assisting a patient, they must systematically **check the patient's identity**, ensure that the treatment corresponds to the prescription, and follow the specific steps indicated in the protocol. These checks, although repetitive, are essential to avoid human error. In addition, protocols often include **checklists** or **double-checking** procedures, which make critical steps such as the preparation of medication or the administration of care to fragile patients even more secure.

When protocols exist, but are not adapted to a specific situation or appear to be ineffective, it is important that caregivers, including orderlies, report these malfunctions. This feedback is essential for adjusting protocols and making them more relevant. For example, a caregiver may report that a hygiene protocol is difficult to apply due to unsuitable equipment or time constraints. By sharing these observations, he or she contributes to the continuous improvement of practices.

Risk and incident management

Risk management in the healthcare environment is an essential dimension of the patient safety culture. It involves anticipating risk situations and implementing strategies to prevent them. This includes infection prevention, medication management, falls prevention, and optimizing patient monitoring. For caregivers, this means being constantly aware of potential risks and adopting proactive behaviors to avoid them.

One example of risk management is the prevention of **nosocomial infections**. Rigorous application of hygiene protocols, such as hand washing and disinfection of surfaces and medical equipment, is crucial to preventing the spread of infections. Caregivers must not only respect these protocols, but also ensure that all staff and patients follow the same rules.

When an incident occurs, the priority is to act immediately to limit its consequences. Next, the incident must be **documented and analyzed** to understand its causes and implement corrective measures. This involves **incident reports**, debriefing meetings and root cause analyses. The aim is to understand why the incident occurred and what systemic failures need to be corrected.

Chapter 9

Interprofessional collaboration and communication

Teamwork in cardiology

○   The caregiver's role in the multidisciplinary team
The caregiver's role in the multidisciplinary team is essential to the smooth running of patient care. The multidisciplinary team is made up of various healthcare professionals, such as doctors, nurses, physiotherapists, psychologists, occupational therapists and many others, each with their own specific skills. In this context, the nursing auxiliary occupies a unique position due to its proximity to the patient, its daily contact and its role in basic care. Their role is complementary to that of other healthcare professionals, contributing to comprehensive, coherent care tailored to the patient's needs.

A key player in daily care

The caregiver is often the person who spends the most time with patients, providing **care for their hygiene, comfort and well-being**, while constantly listening to their needs. This close proximity enables the caregiver to establish a relationship of trust with patients, who feel accompanied and supported on a daily basis. Through simple but essential gestures, such as helping with washing, dressing or mobility, the caregiver contributes directly to the physical and psychological well-being of patients.

The caregiver's role in basic care goes far beyond the technical aspects. He or she is also responsible for carefully observing patients' reactions, behavior and any signs that might indicate a change in their state of health. For example, a change in appetite, unusual fatigue or pain expressed by the patient may be warning signals that the caregiver first notices. This **constant monitoring** enables crucial information to be passed on to the care team, enabling them to adjust care or react rapidly to any deterioration in the patient's condition.

Communication at the heart of collaboration

In a multidisciplinary team, **communication** is one of the cornerstones of collaboration. Each professional has a specific role, but the exchange of information is essential to guarantee continuity and quality of care. As a privileged observer of patients' daily progress, the nursing auxiliary plays a crucial role in **transmitting information**. He or she is often the first to report a change in the patient's condition, be it pain, discomfort, sleep disturbance or mobility problems.

This communication is not limited to nursing care. The caregiver also interacts with other team members, such as physiotherapists, to report mobility problems, or psychologists, to report signs of anxiety or depression in the patient. These interactions are essential for comprehensive care, where physical and psychological care are taken into account in a coordinated fashion.

During consultation meetings, often organized on hospital wards, the caregiver can also provide **valuable information** on the patient's daily life, reaction to care, progress or difficulties. These exchanges enable the whole multidisciplinary team to better understand the patient's needs and adapt interventions accordingly.

Essential support for the nursing team

The nursing auxiliary works under the responsibility of nurses, and their collaboration is a central element in the care process. The caregiver assists the nurse in certain technical tasks, such as taking vital signs, managing medical devices (catheters, infusions), or observing simple clinical signs (temperature, skin color, respiratory rate). They also play an important role in managing comfort care, enabling nurses to concentrate on more technical and specific tasks.

This collaboration between caregiver and nurse is based on **mutual trust** and a clear understanding of each other's roles. Although unable to carry out certain medical procedures, the caregiver is able to monitor the patient on an ongoing basis, and **alert the nurse** if any specific care needs adjusting. In addition, by assisting with procedures such as dressings or patient mobilization, they relieve the nurse's workload while ensuring quality follow-up.

Contributing to patient autonomy

One of the essential roles of the caregiver in the multidisciplinary team is to promote and preserve patient autonomy. In collaboration with physiotherapists and occupational therapists, the caregiver participates in **functional re-education** and accompanies patients in their daily activities. Whether it's encouraging a patient to get up, to walk or to carry out everyday tasks, the caregiver plays an active role in helping them to become more autonomous.

Supporting the patient's autonomy is not limited to the physical aspects. Through regular interaction with patients, caregivers also encourage them to express their needs, make decisions about their own care, and maintain a degree of psychological independence. This support helps to restore the patient's confidence, especially in situations involving post-operative rehabilitation or the management of chronic illnesses.

Psychological and emotional support

The role of the caregiver in a multidisciplinary team is not limited to physical care. It also includes essential **psychological and emotional support**. Faced with illness, hospitalization or dependency, patients often go through moments of anguish, sadness or distress. The caregiver, through his or her constant presence, is often the person to whom the patient will confide. A reassuring word, an attentive ear, or even a simple gesture of comfort can make a big difference to a patient's emotional state.

This emotional support is provided in close collaboration with other professionals, such as psychologists or social workers. When the caregiver detects signs of emotional distress or depression, he or she can refer the patient to these professionals, while ensuring a **benevolent follow-up on** a daily basis. This holistic support is an integral part of quality care, as it enables the whole person to be taken into account, treating not only physical symptoms, but also psychological suffering.

The role of risk prevention

In hospitals and care facilities, risk prevention is a crucial factor in ensuring patient safety. The nursing auxiliary plays a key role in this prevention, whether to avoid falls, prevent nosocomial infections, or monitor the risk of bedsores in bedridden patients. In collaboration with nurses and doctors, they apply **safety protocols** and ensure the implementation of good hygiene and prevention practices.

For example, by ensuring that patients are properly mobilized, that they receive adequate hydration, and that medical devices are maintained to hygienic standards, caregivers help to reduce the risk of complications. His or her role is therefore essential in ensuring that care is carried out in a safe and protocol-compliant environment.

◦　　The importance of care coordination

Care coordination is a fundamental pillar of quality and continuity of care, especially in complex care contexts where several healthcare professionals are involved. It consists in organizing and harmonizing the interventions of the various healthcare professionals around the patient, to ensure an integrated, effective approach focused on individual needs. Care coordination is particularly important in the management of chronic diseases, hospital care, post-operative interventions, and in all situations requiring multidisciplinary collaboration. It is essential not only for patient safety, but also for their well-being and overall experience of care.

Continuity of care: a key factor

One of the main aims of care coordination is to ensure **continuity of care** throughout the patient's healthcare pathway, whether this involves hospitalization, home care or outpatient treatment. Continuity of care ensures that there are no gaps between the different stages of care, guaranteeing that the patient receives coherent care adapted to his or her condition at every stage of the process.

For example, when a patient is hospitalized for surgery, care coordination enables the various stages to be planned: before the operation, during the operation, and after discharge. This includes pre-operative preparation, post-operative care in the intensive care unit, and rehabilitation or care at home. Each of these stages must be perfectly organized and linked to avoid gaps or oversights that could compromise the patient's recovery.

Continuity of care is particularly important in the management of chronic diseases such as diabetes or heart failure. The medical follow-up of these patients requires coordination between the general practitioner, specialists, nurses, and sometimes others such as dieticians or physiotherapists. This synergy between the various players ensures that the patient receives seamless care, and that there are no contradictions between the treatments prescribed by different professionals.

A patient-centred approach

Care coordination places the **patient at the center of the care process**, ensuring that all healthcare professionals work together to meet his or her specific needs. This approach makes it possible to personalize care, taking into account not only the medical aspects, but also the preferences, expectations and realities of each individual patient. This includes, for example, adapting homecare schedules, taking into account patients' treatment preferences, or managing psychological support in the case of serious illnesses.

Care coordination also helps avoid **duplication** or **contradiction** between different treatments or interventions. For example, without proper coordination, a patient could receive conflicting prescriptions from two specialists, which could be detrimental to his or her health or lead to dangerous side effects. Thanks to good coordination, the medical record is shared and updated regularly, providing all those involved with an overview of the patient's care pathway. This makes it possible to adjust treatments as the patient's state of health evolves, and to avoid errors.

Communication: a lever for coordination

Fluid, efficient communication between healthcare professionals is at the heart of care coordination. This communication must be rapid, precise and focused on key information concerning the patient's condition, current treatments and upcoming interventions. To ensure effective coordination, it is essential that every member of the healthcare team is kept informed of medical decisions, test results and changes in the patient's condition.

In a hospital environment, for example, regular exchanges between doctors, nurses, orderlies and other members of the multidisciplinary team are crucial to ensuring that the care provided is consistent and adapted to the patient's situation. Consultative meetings or inter-team communications, where each team member can share his or her observations and adjust care accordingly, are key moments for organizing and coordinating interventions.

Communication with patients and their families is also an essential aspect of care coordination. Patients need to be kept informed of the progress of their condition, the treatments they are being offered, and the different stages in their care. This information enables patients to make informed decisions about their health, and to adopt a proactive stance in their care. Clear, empathetic communication with the patient's loved ones can also facilitate care management, particularly when home interventions are required.

Managing care transitions

The **transition between different care services** is one of the critical moments when effective coordination is essential. Whether it's discharge from hospital to home, transfer between different specialist services, or transition to long-term care, these periods can be sources of confusion or disruption in care if not properly organized.

When a patient leaves hospital to continue care at home, for example, it's important that the homecare nurse receives all relevant information on the patient's condition, the care to be administered, medical prescriptions and recommendations to be followed. This ensures **continuity of care** and avoids complications after discharge. The same principle applies to interdepartmental transfers: if a patient is transferred from intensive care to a rehabilitation department, each team must transmit and receive the information needed to continue treatment.

The management of care transitions often relies on the use of **shared medical records**, which enable each professional to consult the patient's medical history, diagnoses, test results and current treatments. These tools facilitate coordination and help avoid errors linked to poor information transmission.

Preventing errors and complications

Care coordination also plays a fundamental role in preventing medical errors and complications. By ensuring that everyone involved is aware of the care being provided, the treatments being administered and the specific risks associated with the patient's condition, coordination helps minimize the risk of medication errors, inappropriate care or post-operative complications.

A common example is drug interactions. When a patient is under the care of several specialists, he or she may receive prescriptions for drugs that could interact in a harmful way. With proper care coordination, doctors can share information on current treatments and adjust prescriptions accordingly to avoid dangerous interactions.

Similarly, in the case of **patients at high risk of falling**, care coordination enables the implementation of preventive strategies shared by all caregivers. These may include the implementation of safe mobilization protocols, the installation of walking aids, and increased monitoring. These measures, taken in consultation with the care team, help reduce the risk of accidents and complications.

Improving efficiency and patient satisfaction

In addition to guaranteeing better quality of care, coordination also **improves the efficiency** of care. A well-coordinated care team is able to operate more fluidly, reducing the time between interventions and optimizing available resources. This reduces waiting times for patients, avoids redundant or unnecessary care, and makes better use of the skills of each healthcare professional.

Patient satisfaction is also enhanced when they feel that their care is well organized and that healthcare professionals communicate seamlessly with each other. A patient who sees that his or her care is well coordinated, that each professional knows his or her file and that he or she benefits from continuity of care, is more inclined to trust the healthcare team and feel secure. This satisfaction also contributes to **patient compliance**, as a well-informed and well-supported patient is more likely to follow prescribed treatments correctly.

◦ Concrete examples of effective collaboration

Effective collaboration between different healthcare professionals is essential to delivering quality patient care and ensuring comprehensive, coherent and personalized care. Here are a few concrete examples of how successful collaboration between care assistants, nurses, doctors, physiotherapists and other members of the multidisciplinary team can significantly improve the quality of care and patient safety.

Example 1: Managing a patient undergoing rehabilitation after a fracture

Imagine a patient hospitalized after a hip fracture, requiring surgery followed by a period of rehabilitation. In this case, collaboration between orderlies, nurses, doctors and physiotherapists is crucial to ensure optimal recovery.

The role of the nursing auxiliary: On a day-to-day basis, the caregiver assists the patient with hygiene care, transfers between bed and chair, and moving around the room or hospital corridors. He or she helps to fit compression stockings to prevent thrombosis and to prevent bedsores in this patient with reduced mobility. The caregiver also observes signs of discomfort or pain in the patient during mobilizations, and reports them to the team.

Role of the physiotherapist: Every day, the physiotherapist helps the patient to gradually regain his or her mobility through appropriate exercises. He or she may, for example, work with the patient on walking re-education, ensuring that he or she learns to use crutches or a walker correctly.

Collaboration: Collaboration between the physiotherapist and the caregiver is essential. The caregiver assists the physiotherapist by mobilizing the patient before or after rehabilitation sessions, and by helping to prepare mobilization exercises. Thanks to this daily interaction, the caregiver can inform the physiotherapist of the patient's progress or difficulties, such as persistent pain or unusual stiffness, so that exercises and the pace of rehabilitation can be adjusted.

The nurse's role: The nurse manages post-surgical medical aspects, such as monitoring dressings, signs of infection and post-operative pain. He or she adjusts analgesic treatments according to the nursing auxiliary's observations and the physiotherapist's feedback on the patient's progress.

In this case, effective collaboration between the caregiver, physiotherapist and nurse ensures fluid rehabilitation tailored to the patient's needs, while regularly monitoring progress and making any necessary adjustments.

Example 2: Managing a hypoglycemic crisis in a diabetic patient

Let's take the example of a diabetic patient hospitalized for another pathology. One morning, while checking vital signs, the orderly observes that the patient is particularly weak, confused and sweating excessively. He suspected hypoglycemia.

Role of the caregiver : The caregiver, trained to recognize the signs of hypoglycemia, immediately measures the patient's glucose level using a glucometer. The result indicates a very low blood sugar level. He or she quickly alerts the nurse, while ensuring that the patient is comfortable and safe, to avoid falls due to confusion.

The nurse's role: Once informed, the nurse intervenes rapidly, administering an appropriate treatment to raise the sugar level (such as sugar gel or a glucagon injection if necessary). He or she then monitors the patient to ensure that his or her condition stabilizes.

The doctor's role: The nurse informs the doctor of the incident. He reviews the patient's treatment to adjust the insulin dose or modify the dietary plan, in order to prevent possible hypoglycemia relapses.

Collaboration: In this example, collaboration between the caregiver, nurse and doctor enabled the rapid identification of a risky situation, immediate intervention to stabilize the patient, and a review of care to avoid further complications. The caregiver's initial observation, relayed to the nurse and doctor, illustrates how good communication and a clear division of roles can ensure patient safety.

Example 3: Accompanying a palliative care patient

Another example concerns a terminally ill cancer patient, admitted to a palliative care unit to relieve pain and improve quality of life at the end of the course. This type of situation calls for close collaboration between the various members of the care team: doctors, nurses, care assistants, psychologists and sometimes chaplains or social workers.

The caregiver's role : The caregiver provides hygiene care, ensures patient comfort, regularly adjusts the patient's position to prevent pressure sores, and monitors for signs of pain or discomfort. They are also often the patient's confidant, able to listen to their anxieties, fears and needs.

The nurse's role: The nurse is in charge of administering medical care, such as infusions, painkillers or sedatives. He/she adjusts doses according to the doctor's instructions and the observations of the nursing auxiliary.

The doctor's role: The doctor decides on the care plan and the treatments to be administered to relieve pain. He or she works closely with nurses and care assistants to adapt painkiller doses to the patient's changing needs.

Role of the psychologist and chaplain: The psychologist supports the patient and family in dealing with the emotional and psychological suffering associated with the end-of-life stage. Depending on the patient's beliefs, the chaplain can also offer spiritual support.

Collaboration: The entire team meets regularly to discuss the patient's progress, emotional and physical needs, and to adjust the care plan. Thanks to the valuable information provided by the caregiver on the patient's day-to-day condition, the doctor and nurse can adjust treatments accordingly, while the psychologist or chaplain provides the necessary psychological and spiritual support. This collaboration enables us to offer comprehensive, personalized support to patients at the end of life, in a calm, respectful environment.

Example 4: Discharge from hospital and follow-up at home

When patients are discharged from hospital after prolonged hospitalization for heart failure, collaboration between the hospital and homecare services is crucial to ensure continuity of care.

Role of the hospital orderly: Before the patient is discharged, the hospital orderly works with the team to prepare the patient to return home. They ensure that the patient understands care instructions, knows how to manage daily activities and is aware of warning signs of complications.

Role of the hospital nurse: The hospital nurse ensures that all necessary medical information (treatment, post-operative care, home monitoring) is transmitted to the homecare service.

The homecare nurse's role: Once the patient has returned home, the homecare nurse takes over to monitor the patient's state of health, administer treatments and manage medical devices (infusions, catheters, etc.).

Collaboration: The transfer of information between hospital teams and homecare workers helps to avoid breaks in the continuity of care, and ensures that the patient is properly cared for as soon as he or she returns home. The home care assistant, who regularly provides basic and comfort care, can communicate with the nurse in the event of a problem, and help him or her to adjust care as the situation evolves.

These concrete examples show how **effective collaboration** between different healthcare professionals ensures comprehensive, safe care tailored to patients' needs. Each member of the team brings valuable expertise and observation to the table, and it is thanks to this complementarity and fluid communication that patients benefit from quality care, whether in hospital or at home. By working closely together, caregivers can anticipate problems, adjust treatments and support the patient's care journey, while ensuring his or her physical, emotional and psychological well-being.

Communication with patients and their families

　　　　◦　　Communication techniques for cardiac patients
Communication techniques adapted to cardiac patients play a fundamental role in the quality of care and well-being of patients. Heart disease is often a source of anxiety, uncertainty and sometimes emotional distress for patients and their families. Clear, empathetic communication tailored to patients' specific needs not only reduces their stress, but also improves their understanding of their condition, actively involves them in their care, and promotes adherence to treatment. In this context, the nursing auxiliary, in direct and regular contact with patients, must develop communication techniques that combine competence and humanity.

Take into account your emotional and psychological state

Heart patients, especially those facing events such as myocardial infarction, surgery or a diagnosis of heart failure, can be **emotionally charged**. These heart conditions often trigger feelings of vulnerability, anxiety about the future, and sometimes even fear of death. In this context, the caregiver needs to be an **attentive** and empathetic listener, taking the time to take an interest in the patient's feelings.

It's important to create a **safe space** for **communication**, where patients feel free to express their concerns without judgment. For example, when a patient expresses fear about an imminent operation, the caregiver must listen carefully, validating the patient's emotions ("I understand that this may worry you"), while providing reassuring answers based on medical information. It is often useful to rephrase what the patient is saying, to show that his or her words have been understood ("You're afraid the operation will be risky, aren't you?"). This makes the patient feel listened to and taken seriously.

Adapting language to the patient's comprehension

Simplicity and clarity are essential when communicating with cardiac patients. Often complex medical terms can make patients feel confused or powerless. It is therefore essential to adapt the vocabulary used so that it is accessible to all, without infantilizing the patient.

For example, instead of talking about a "coronary angiogram", the caregiver can simply explain that this is an examination to visualize the heart's arteries, to check for blockages. By explaining care or treatment in simple terms, patients feel more confident and better informed, which helps them to actively participate in their care.

The use of **metaphors** or concrete examples can also facilitate understanding of complex concepts. For example, to explain the placement of a stent, the caregiver may compare the blocked artery to a clogged pipe, and the stent to a small spring that keeps the pipe open to allow blood to flow normally. This approach makes explanations more accessible and engaging for the patient.

Encouraging active patient participation

Active patient participation in treatment is a key factor in the success of cardiac care. A well-informed and involved patient will be better able to follow his or her treatment correctly, modify his or her lifestyle if necessary, and recognize the warning signs of a heart problem.

To achieve this, the caregiver must encourage the patient to ask questions, express doubts and participate in decisions concerning his or her health. For example, when explaining what medication to take after cardiac surgery, it is useful to ask the patient if he or she has understood the instructions and if he or she has any questions. By inviting patients to express themselves, caregivers encourage them to take an active role in managing their health, rather than passively enduring care.

In cases where the patient needs to adopt new lifestyle habits (such as an adapted diet or regular physical activity), the caregiver can use **open-ended questions** to initiate discussion: "How do you plan to integrate these changes into your daily life?" or "What difficulties do you expect to encounter with this treatment?". This participatory approach helps patients to feel more autonomous and to better understand the implications of their treatment.

Reducing anxiety through non-verbal communication

Non-verbal communication is a crucial element in the management of cardiac patients. Tone of voice, facial expressions, posture and eye contact play a fundamental role in how the message is perceived by the patient. A smile, a reassuring look or an open posture can help reduce patient anxiety, create a climate of trust and encourage exchange.

It's important to be **present and attentive**. By actively listening to the patient, maintaining eye contact and avoiding any form of distraction (such as looking at a screen or consulting papers), the caregiver shows the patient that he or she is fully available to him or her. This attention to the patient can reassure him/her that his/her concerns are being taken into account.

Supportive gestures, such as placing a hand on the patient's shoulder or adjusting a pillow for comfort, reinforce the feeling of security and caring. This allows the patient to feel surrounded and supported during an often anxious period.

Adapting communication to patients in distress

Cardiac patients can sometimes experience physical or emotional distress, for example during a heart attack or acute complication. In these critical moments, it's important to maintain clear, **reassuring** communication, while adopting a firm, calm tone.

When a patient is in distress, the caregiver's first reaction should be to reassure them that they are being looked after. Simple, soothing phrases such as "We're here, we'll take care of you" can help reduce panic. It's also crucial to give brief, precise information: "I'll take your blood pressure now" or "We'll call the doctor". This helps to keep the patient informed of what's going on, without further distressing them.

In these moments, the use of a **calm, collected tone of voice** is essential to reassure the patient, even if the situation is serious. Maintaining a certain consistency in gesture and tone helps to create an atmosphere of control and security, enabling the patient to remain as calm as possible.

Involving family and friends in communication

Heart disease affects not only patients, but also their families and loved ones, who may feel anxious about the evolution of the patient's state of health. The caregiver also plays a role in **communicating with loved ones**, providing them with clear information adapted to their level of understanding, while supporting them emotionally.

Involving loved ones in communication helps prepare them for home care, for changes in the patient's lifestyle, and for recognizing warning signs. For example, explaining to loved ones what to do in the event of chest pain, or how to encourage the patient to adopt a healthier diet, is a way of including them in the care process and reassuring them about the patient's overall care.

○ Managing families' expectations and emotions

Managing the expectations and emotions of families is a crucial component of caregivers' work, particularly in complex or delicate medical contexts such as cardiology departments. Families, like patients, often experience moments of uncertainty, anxiety and sometimes distress when faced with the illness or hospitalization of a loved one. The caregiver, in direct contact with the patient and family, plays a key role in managing expectations, calming emotions and conveying information in a clear and reassuring way. Empathetic, appropriate communication is therefore essential to support families and foster a serene environment conducive to the patient's recovery.

Understanding family emotions

The families of patients, particularly those with serious heart disease, experience **intense** emotions that can range from worry and frustration to fear, anger and despair. These emotions are often exacerbated by uncertainty about the course of the disease, fear of losing a loved one or difficulty in understanding complex medical terms. In the face of this, it's crucial for the caregiver to **listen attentively** and recognize the legitimacy of these feelings.

For example, a family who learns that their loved one's state of health requires major surgery, such as coronary bypass, may react with anxiety, even anguish. In this context, the caregiver must first and foremost understand the source of these emotions: fear of the operation, stress linked to hospitalization, or lack of understanding of the risks and benefits of the procedure.

Active listening and empathic communication

One of the first steps in dealing with families' emotions is to practice **active listening**. This means being fully present, without interrupting or judging, while allowing relatives to share their fears, doubts or frustrations. By listening attentively, the caregiver shows the family that their emotions are heard and respected. This process of listening not only calms loved ones, but also identifies the real concerns behind their emotions.

The caregiver can rephrase what family members are saying to make sure they feel understood: "You seem very anxious about the operation. Is it the fear of risk that worries you most? This rephrasing opens up a more constructive dialogue and helps the family to clarify their expectations or concerns.

Empathetic communication is also essential for calming families. It involves acknowledging their emotions while reassuring them: "I understand that this situation is difficult for you. Your concern is completely normal, and please know that we are doing everything we can to take care of your loved one". By adopting a calm, caring and sincere tone, the caregiver can reduce families' anxiety and make them feel that they are not alone in dealing with their loved one's illness.

Providing clear, appropriate information

One of the major challenges for families is often to **understand** the patient's medical situation, especially when dealing with complex diseases such as heart disease. Medical terms, surgical procedures and prognoses can be difficult for the uninitiated to grasp. One of the caregiver's essential missions is therefore to **translate** this information into simple, understandable terms, while remaining transparent about the patient's state of health.

It's important to adapt the way information is provided to the family's ability to assimilate it. Some families may prefer precise technical information, while others will need more general explanations. For example, if the family asks for details of a drug treatment, the caregiver can explain in simple terms: "This medicine helps relax the arteries of the heart to improve blood circulation". Giving clear, accessible information reduces misunderstanding and helps families feel more in control of the situation.

Caregivers also need to be **transparent** and reassuring at the same time. This means not downplaying risks or offering false assurances, but rather presenting reality in an understandable way. If the patient is going through a critical phase, it's essential to explain this honestly to the family, while informing them of the steps being taken to ensure the best possible treatment: "It's true that the situation is delicate at the moment, but we're monitoring his condition closely and the doctors are taking all the necessary measures to stabilize his situation".

Manage expectations realistically

Another key component of family management is **managing expectations**. Some families may expect a rapid recovery or return to normal, even in situations where the prognosis is uncertain or recovery is lengthy. In such cases, it's important to explain the various stages of treatment and recovery, while ensuring that expectations are realistic.

For example, for a patient who has undergone major heart surgery, it's crucial to remind families that recovery can be slow, and that there may be phases of fatigue, rehabilitation and post-operative monitoring. The caregiver may say: "After such an operation, it's normal for recovery to take several weeks. We'll do everything we can to help him through this phase, but it's important not to rush.

In some cases, it can be difficult for the family to accept a gloomier prognosis, especially when palliative or end-of-life care is involved. Here, the caregiver plays a key role in **preparing the family** for this reality, working in concert with the medical team and psychologists. Managing expectations at these moments relies on a **delicate balance** between compassion and clarity, respecting families' right to be informed while supporting them emotionally.

Providing emotional and practical support

In times of crisis or concern for a sick loved one, families need **emotional support**. This can include simple gestures, such as offering a space to rest, a warm drink, or just being present to listen without judgment. The caregiver, as the person they trust on a daily basis, can play an important role in this support. Sometimes, it's not just a matter of talking, but of **being there** for the family, offering a sense of security at a difficult time.

Beyond emotional support, it may also be necessary to offer **practical support**. This may involve answering logistical questions (visiting schedules, information on home care after discharge) or guiding the family through administrative procedures. By addressing these practical concerns, the caregiver can lighten the mental load on families, who are often overwhelmed by managing the practical aspects associated with hospitalization.

Involving the family in care

Whenever possible, **involving the family in care** can not only strengthen the bond between patient and loved ones, but also reassure the family about the quality of care. Caregivers can encourage relatives to take part in simple tasks, such as helping the patient eat or accompanying him/her in mobilization exercises. This allows the family to feel useful and actively involved in their loved one's recovery.

Involving the family in care also means giving them the tools they need to **assume certain** responsibilities **after** discharge from hospital, particularly in home care. The caregiver can explain what needs to be done, such as monitoring for signs of complication, taking medication or taking precautions. This helps relatives prepare for the transition out of hospital, and reinforces their sense of competence.

○ Facilitating shared decision-making

Facilitating shared decision-making is an essential approach in patient-centered care, particularly in the medical field. It involves the patient, and sometimes the patient's family, in the decision-making process concerning care, treatment and therapeutic options. It is based on an open and respectful dialogue between caregivers and patients, enabling the latter to fully understand the implications of each option, and to actively participate in the choice of care that corresponds to their preferences, values and life situation. The caregiver plays a key role in this dynamic, as a privileged and close contact with the patient.

Understanding shared decision-making

Shared decision-making is a collaborative process in which patients and caregivers work together to choose the most appropriate treatment or care. This model of care marks an important shift in the relationship between caregiver and patient, emphasizing a **collaborative** rather than directive approach. Rather than receiving instructions from doctors or nurses, patients are invited to express their preferences, ask questions and co-construct, with the care team, the decisions that concern them.

This approach is particularly important in the context of **chronic diseases**, such as heart disease, where patients are often faced with complex choices, particularly concerning long-term treatments, lifestyle changes or surgical interventions. By actively involving patients, caregivers help them to better understand the issues at stake and make informed choices, which can improve therapeutic compliance and patient satisfaction with their care.

Making information clear and accessible

One of the caregiver's fundamental roles in the shared decision-making process is to **facilitate understanding of the** treatment options available. Patients may feel overwhelmed by complex medical terms or by the amount of technical information they are given. The caregiver must therefore translate this information into clear, accessible language.

For example, if a heart patient has to choose between medication and surgery, the caregiver can explain the advantages and disadvantages of each option in simple language: "If you choose medication, it may help reduce symptoms without surgery, but it will require regular monitoring and may have side effects. Surgery could resolve the problem more definitively, but there are risks associated with surgery".

Clarifying options enables patients to better understand what's at stake, to ask questions and discuss their preferences, without being paralyzed by uncertainty or fear of choosing wrong. This transparency fosters an open dialogue between patient and healthcare team.

Encouraging the expression of patient preferences

In a shared decision-making process, it is essential that the patient feels **listened to** and encouraged to express his or her preferences, concerns and expectations. The caregiver, often in regular and prolonged contact with the patient, can play a key role in encouraging this expression. He or she can, for example, ask open-ended questions that invite the patient to share his or her thoughts: "How do you feel about these options?", "Is there anything that worries you about the treatment?" or "Do you have any preferences about how you would like to be cared for?".

By enabling the patient to verbalize his or her preferences, the caregiver helps to make the patient a player in his or her own health. This can also help the medical team to better understand the patient's priorities and adapt the care plan accordingly. For example, a patient may express a preference for a treatment that enables him or her to maintain a certain degree of autonomy or a particular lifestyle. The care team can then take this information into account to propose an approach that respects these wishes.

Support decision-making in moments of doubt

Some patients may find it difficult to make a decision, especially when the options involve risk or uncertainty. In these cases, the caregiver can help **clarify the issues**, breaking down information into simpler steps, while offering emotional support. An indecisive patient can be encouraged to take the time needed to think things through, ask further questions or discuss concerns with family.

The caregiver can also remind the patient that the decision doesn't have to be made immediately, if time permits, and that it's normal to need more information or time to reflect. This can help alleviate the pressure felt by the patient when faced with a difficult choice, by giving them the space they need to make an informed and serene decision.

Involving the family in decision-making

In many cases, especially when the patient is vulnerable or elderly, the **family** plays an important role in the decision-making process. The caregiver can facilitate communication between the patient, the family and the healthcare team, ensuring that everyone understands the options and implications of the choices to be made. Sometimes, the family may hold values and preferences that the patient is reluctant to express alone, or conversely, they can be a crucial support in helping the patient clarify his or her expectations.

The caregiver can encourage constructive discussion by facilitating respectful dialogue between all parties. For example, if a patient is hesitating between two treatments, but the family is concerned about the risks of surgery, the caregiver can propose a **consultation meeting** with the doctor, patient and family to discuss the best options together, while respecting the patient's wishes. This collaborative approach helps avoid tensions or misunderstandings, and ensures that the final decision is well understood and accepted by all.

Ensuring informed decision-making

For the shared decision-making process to be truly effective, it is crucial to ensure that the patient makes an **informed decision**, i.e. that he or she fully understands the **benefits, risks and alternatives** of each proposed option. The caregiver, in conjunction with the medical team, must ensure that the patient has all the information required to make an informed choice.

This involves checking that the patient has understood the information given, and answering all questions clearly and transparently. If any questions remain unanswered, the caregiver can refer the patient to a doctor or specialist who can provide more precise answers. Similarly, if the patient wishes to make a decision contrary to medical advice, it is important to respect this choice, as long as it is based on a full understanding of the implications.

Encouraging autonomy and respect for patient values

Finally, facilitating shared decision-making also means encouraging **respect for the** patient's **values and priorities**. Each individual has his or her own beliefs, preferences and expectations concerning the way in which he or she wishes to be cared for. Some patients may prefer a more proactive approach, with aggressive treatments to maximize their chances of recovery, while others may prioritize **quality of life** and choose less invasive treatments, even if this reduces their chances of survival.

The caregiver must listen to these values and ensure that they are respected in the care process. For example, a patient at the end of life may prefer palliative care to intensive treatment, and it is essential that this preference is not only heard, but also respected by the entire care team. The caregiver can play a mediating role by reminding the team of the patient's expressed wishes, and ensuring that these choices are taken into account in treatment decisions.

Managing conflict and stress within the team

      °   Identifying and resolving workplace conflicts
Identifying and resolving conflict in the workplace is an essential skill for maintaining a healthy and productive working environment, especially in such demanding fields as healthcare. Conflicts can arise for a variety of reasons: misunderstandings, differences of opinion, communication problems or the pressures of professional responsibilities. When these conflicts are not

identified and managed quickly, they can lead to tension within the team, a deterioration in the quality of care and a decline in well-being at work. The caregiver, in daily contact with other team members, plays a crucial role in conflict prevention and resolution.

Identifying sources of conflict

Before resolving a conflict, it's essential to know how to **identify** its **sources**. Conflicts in the workplace can be relational, organizational or linked to differences in the way responsibilities are handled. Here are some of the most common causes of conflict in the healthcare sector:

1. **Communication problems**: Misunderstandings or poor transmission of information between colleagues can lead to errors, frustration and a sense of injustice. For example, if care instructions are not clearly explained or misinterpreted, this can generate tension between caregivers.

2. **Uneven workload**: The feeling that some team members are carrying a heavier load than others can lead to frustration. When the distribution of tasks is not perceived as fair, conflicts can arise over responsibilities.

3. **Different personalities or working styles**: Caregivers often come from a variety of backgrounds, with different ways of working and reacting. Sometimes, these differences can lead to disagreements or friction.

4. **Lack of recognition**: Another common cause of conflict is **lack of recognition**. When team members feel that their work or efforts are not recognized, this can lead to feelings of frustration or injustice.

5. **Stress and fatigue**: Hospitals are high-pressure environments, and accumulated stress and fatigue can

amplify minor tensions. Under stress, a minor disagreement can quickly escalate into open conflict.

Recognizing warning signs

Conflict doesn't always manifest itself immediately and openly. It often begins with **subtle signs**, such as reduced communication, avoidance behaviour, or changes in relations between colleagues (refusal to collaborate, latent tensions). As a close member of the care team, the caregiver is well placed to observe these signals. It is essential to remain alert to these signs in order to prevent conflict from escalating.

For example, if a team member becomes more distant or adopts a dry tone in his or her exchanges, this may indicate unease. Similarly, if discussions become more tense, with defensive responses or indirect criticism, this is a sign that conflict is developing. **Recognizing these signs** early on can help defuse the situation before it escalates.

ave.

Resolving conflicts through communication

Open, caring communication is the key to resolving conflict. When a conflict arises, it is essential to create a space where each person can express his or her point of view without being judged. This requires an **active listening attitude**: listening to what each person has to say, without interrupting, and rephrasing to ensure that the message has been understood. This helps to clarify misunderstandings and identify the needs or concerns of each party.

The caregiver can act as an **intermediary**, facilitating dialogue between people in conflict. For example, if two colleagues are arguing about the distribution of tasks, the caregiver can propose an open discussion where everyone can explain their feelings. In such cases, it is important to remain neutral and not to take sides, but rather to guide the conversation towards constructive solutions.

Assertiveness is also a key skill in conflict resolution. It means expressing needs or disagreements clearly, respectfully and without aggression. For example, if a caregiver feels that the workload is unfair, he or she might say: "I sometimes feel overloaded and would like to discuss the distribution of tasks to see how we can organize ourselves better together". This approach enables problems to be formulated constructively, without accusing or blaming the other person.

Finding joint solutions

Once each party has expressed its point of view, the aim is to **find common solutions** that suit everyone. This often involves **compromise**, with each party agreeing to take a step towards the other to re-establish a balance. For example, if the conflict concerns the distribution of tasks, the team can review the organization of work and draw up a new schedule that takes everyone's constraints into account.

The caregiver can suggest **concrete solutions** that meet everyone's needs. For example, if the problem concerns a lack of communication between team members, it may be suggested to set up **regular meetings** or moments of formal exchange to improve the transmission of information. These initiatives help to reduce sources of misunderstanding and foster a calmer working climate.

It's important that the solutions adopted are **realistic and workable**. Sometimes, resolving a conflict involves small adjustments, such as better organization of care or clarification of everyone's roles. Follow-up on decisions taken is also essential to ensure that tensions do not recur in the future.

Preventing conflict: creating a culture of respect and collaboration

The best way to resolve conflict is to **avoid** it in the first place, by creating a work environment where respect, collaboration and communication are central values. In the care environment, where stress and pressure are often present, it is crucial to promote a **culture of mutual support** and recognition.

Encouraging regular exchanges within the team, whether through team meetings or informal moments, helps to **anticipate frustrations** and tackle problems before they become sources of conflict. What's more, highlighting everyone's efforts and valuing teamwork fosters a positive climate, where everyone feels recognized in their role.

Conflict management training can also be a proactive solution to better prepare teams to deal with disagreements. Learning to recognize the signs of incipient conflict, to use assertive communication techniques, and to handle situations calmly and rationally can help defuse tensions before they escalate.

Managing emotions and reacting calmly

Emotions often play a central role in conflict. Anger, frustration or a sense of injustice can amplify tensions. It is therefore crucial to learn how to manage one's own emotions, but also to recognize those of others. When a colleague is angry or upset, the caregiver must be **calm and patient**, and avoid responding in the same tone. The ability to **defuse emotions** by remaining calm and offering a space for peaceful dialogue is essential to prevent conflict from escalating.

If emotions are too strong for constructive discussion at the moment, it can be helpful to **step back** and offer to resume the conversation once everyone has regained their composure. This avoids impulsive words or actions that could escalate the conflict.

○ Non-violent communication strategies

Non-violent communication (NVC) is a communication approach based on empathy, benevolence and mutual understanding. It aims to establish a respectful and constructive dialogue, even in situations of tension or disagreement. This method, developed by Marshall Rosenberg, is based on the idea that each person, by clearly expressing his or her needs and listening to the needs of others, can defuse conflict and foster more harmonious relationships. In the workplace, particularly in healthcare, adopting non-violent communication can improve exchanges between colleagues, strengthen collaboration within teams and prevent conflict, while promoting a better quality of life at work.

The fundamental principles of non-violent communication

Non-violent communication is based on four essential principles: **observation**, **expression of feelings**, **identification of needs** and **formulation of clear requests**. These principles, fluidly applied, help to foster respectful, constructive dialogue.

1. **Observation**: The first step in NVC is to observe the facts objectively, without judgment or interpretation. It involves describing the situation as it is, without making criticisms or accusations. For example, if a colleague arrives late for a meeting, instead of saying "You're always late, that's disrespectful", we could say "Today, you arrived 20 minutes after the meeting started".

2. **Feelings**: The second step is to express how you feel about the situation you've observed, using precise terms to describe your emotions. It's important not to accuse the other person of provoking these emotions, but to focus on how you feel. For example, "I feel frustrated and stressed when the meeting doesn't start on time".

3. **Needs**: Next, NVC invites us to identify the needs behind these feelings. This helps us to understand why a situation affects us the way it does. For example: "I need meetings to start on time so that we can keep to our schedule and work efficiently".

4. **Request**: The final step is to formulate a concrete, positive and realistic request to improve the situation or meet the needs expressed. The idea is not to give orders, but to invite the other person to cooperate. For example: "Would it be possible for us to start the next meeting on time, or to agree on a more suitable time together?

These four steps, followed in a fluid and respectful way, help **defuse tensions** by promoting empathy, listening and clarity in exchanges. They offer a simple yet powerful framework for improving the quality of interactions in sometimes stressful or tense work environments.

Using empathy to foster mutual understanding

One of the pillars of non-violent communication **is empathy**, i.e. the ability to put oneself in another person's shoes to understand their feelings and needs. By developing this skill, we can better understand our interlocutor's feelings and react more appropriately.

For example, in a care setting, if a colleague seems irritated or tense, empathy helps us to perceive that his or her behavior may be linked to fatigue, pressure or personal concerns, rather than a deliberate desire to create tension. By recognizing this reality, we can adopt a more benevolent attitude and avoid responding aggressively or taking things personally.

To foster empathy, it's important to **pay attention to non-verbal** signals (facial expressions, tone of voice, posture), which often reveal how the other person is feeling, even if they don't express their emotions directly. Active listening is also essential: this means paying full attention to what the other person is saying, without interrupting or trying to formulate an immediate response. By rephrasing the other person's words to check that you've understood ("If I understand correctly, do you feel under pressure because of the workload?"), you show that you're paying attention and seeking to understand, which reinforces dialogue and openness.

Practicing self-empathy to better manage emotions

In non-violent communication, it's also important to cultivate **self-empathy**: this consists in recognizing and accepting our own emotions, without judging or repressing them. By being more attuned to our needs and feelings, we're better equipped to handle stressful or conflictual situations with calm and clarity.

When we're stressed or overwhelmed by our emotions, it's easy to react impulsively or defensively. By taking a moment to practice self-empathy, we can acknowledge how we feel, identify our unmet needs, and choose a more constructive way of approaching the situation. For example, if a colleague's remark hurts our feelings, we can take a moment to say to ourselves: "I feel hurt because I need respect and recognition in my work". By identifying the source of our emotion, we are then better able to communicate our feelings in a non-violent and respectful way.

Self-empathy is also essential to avoid emotional exhaustion in demanding work environments. By regularly taking the time to connect with our own emotions and needs, we can better regulate stress and maintain a healthier emotional balance.

Express disagreements without aggression

In the workplace, it's natural for **disagreements** to arise, whether over decisions, work methods or priorities. Non-violent communication is a way of expressing disagreement without offending or hurting the other person, while maintaining a dynamic of dialogue and cooperation.

When expressing disagreement, it's important to stay **focused on the facts** and avoid accusations or generalizations. For example, instead of saying: "You never pay attention to others", it would be more effective to say: "I noticed that at our last meeting, you didn't take the team's suggestions into account". Then, by expressing your **feelings** and **needs**, you can avoid putting the other person in a defensive position: "I felt frustrated because I needed my ideas to be listened to and taken into account".

Finally, it's useful to formulate a **constructive request** to improve the situation in the future: "Would it be possible for us to take more time at the next meeting to discuss everyone's proposals? This approach allows disagreement to be expressed respectfully, opening the door to cooperation rather than confrontation.

Handling criticism with kindness

In the workplace, it's not uncommon to receive **criticism**, whether constructive or not. Non-violent communication offers an approach for receiving criticism more calmly, and avoiding aggressive or defensive reactions.

When we receive criticism, it's important to remember that it often expresses an **unsatisfied need** or feeling of the other person. Rather than seeing it as a personal attack, we can try to understand what's behind the criticism. For example, if a colleague says: "You're always late with your reports", we can try to understand the need behind this remark: "You seem frustrated by report deadlines. Do you need to be more punctual to meet deadlines?

This attitude of openness helps to defuse tensions and turn criticism into an opportunity to improve communication and collaboration.

Formulate clear, respectful requests

A central aspect of non-violent communication is the ability to **formulate clear**, realistic and respectful requests, in order to solve a problem or improve a situation. Requests must be precise, positive (formulated in terms of actions to be accomplished, rather than what the other should stop doing), and respectful of the other's autonomy.

Rather than making **demands**, which can provoke resistance, the idea is to propose **collaborative solutions**. For example, if a colleague has a tendency to interrupt meetings, instead of saying "You've got to stop interrupting", we can formulate a positive request: "Would it be possible to go around the table so that everyone can express themselves without being interrupted?". This approach paves the way for respectful dialogue and the search for compromise.

- ○ The importance of active listening and constructive feedback

Active listening and **constructive feedback** are two fundamental pillars for effective, caring communication in any working environment, but especially in environments where human interaction is central, such as the healthcare sector. These two skills enhance the quality of exchanges between colleagues, strengthen team cohesion, promote personal and professional development, and guarantee a climate of trust and mutual respect. Active listening and constructive feedback are not just communication tools, but approaches that value people, create authentic dialogue, and contribute to problem-solving and collective growth.

The importance of active listening

Active listening is much more than just listening. It involves being fully present and attentive when another person expresses themselves, seeking to understand not only the words, but also the emotions, intentions and needs underlying the discourse. It requires complete attention, free from judgments or interruptions, in order to create a space where the interlocutor feels heard, understood and respected. In a work environment, especially in healthcare, where human interaction is frequent and crucial, active listening helps to prevent misunderstandings, improve the quality of care and strengthen professional relationships.

Active listening is based on several key elements:

1. **Total presence**: Being genuinely available to the other person, without distractions. This involves maintaining eye contact, adopting an open posture and avoiding consulting your phone or thinking about other things. In a hospital setting, where caregivers are often overworked, active listening requires a conscious effort to make time for each person, whether colleague or patient.

2. **Verbal and non-verbal reactions**: Non-verbal signals (nods, smiles, facial expressions) and verbal signals ("I see", "I understand") show that you're paying close attention to what's being said. These signs, subtle though they may be, tell the speaker that his or her words are being taken into account. For example, when a caregiver listens to a patient or colleague expressing a problem, his or her non-verbal reactions make the person feel understood and reassured.

3. **Rephrasing and clarification**: To make sure you've understood what the other person has said, it's useful to rephrase what they've said, for example: "If I understand correctly, you're feeling stressed by the workload this week, aren't you? This technique not only verifies that the message has been well received, but also shows that you attach importance to what has been said.

4. **Empathy**: Active listening also means trying to put yourself in the other person's shoes, understanding not

only their words, but also their emotions. It's about recognizing the feelings behind the words, which strengthens the bond with the interlocutor and facilitates dialogue. For example, if a colleague expresses annoyance, active listening helps to understand that this annoyance may be the result of fatigue or stress, and not a personal attack.

Active listening is therefore a powerful tool for **defusing tensions**, improving professional relations and ensuring a better understanding of expectations and needs. It fosters a climate of respect and trust, essential for harmonious collaboration.

The benefits of active listening in the workplace

Active listening, while requiring time and energy, produces many benefits, especially in a work environment such as healthcare, where coordination and communication are essential.

1. **Reducing misunderstandings**: By actively listening, caregivers ensure that the information exchanged is clearly understood. This helps to avoid errors in patient care or in the allocation of tasks. For example, by rephrasing what a doctor or nurse has asked, the caregiver ensures that instructions are properly applied.

2. **Improved relationships**: When people feel listened to and understood, they are more likely to collaborate and invest in teamwork. Active listening thus strengthens cohesion and understanding within teams, creating a more serene and cooperative working environment.

3. **Confidence-building**: A staff member or patient who feels listened to is more inclined to trust the other person. This is particularly important in caregiver-patient relationships, where trust is a key factor in the healing process and adherence to treatment.

4. **Quick problem solving**: By actively listening to your colleagues' problems or frustrations, you're more likely to find solutions quickly and constructively. Listening helps to identify the real causes of conflicts or difficulties, and to respond appropriately.

The importance of constructive feedback

Constructive feedback is the other component of effective communication. It helps to improve performance, correct mistakes and encourage good practice. Constructive feedback, when given in a benevolent and precise manner, not only **helps the other person to progress**, but also strengthens the professional relationship by creating a space for mutual exchange and learning.

Effective feedback must be :

1. **Specific**: It's essential to avoid generalizations ("You always do it wrong") and focus on concrete, observable facts. For example, instead of saying "You don't get involved enough", it's more effective to say: "At the last meeting, you remained silent even though we needed your opinion on the organization of care".

2. **Future-oriented**: Constructive feedback should not only point out what went wrong, but suggest solutions for the future. It's important to guide the person towards concrete improvements: "Next time, it would be helpful if you could share your ideas at the start of the meeting, so that we can incorporate your suggestions".

3. **Respectful and caring**: The tone and manner of giving feedback are as important as the message itself. It's

essential to remain respectful and not judge or criticize the person, but rather their actions. The aim is to encourage the other person to progress, not to blame or humiliate them. For example, instead of saying "You're really disorganized", you could say "I've noticed that certain tasks haven't been prioritized, and this has created delays. I think we could improve organization by prioritizing tasks".

4. **Balanced**: Good feedback doesn't have to be exclusively negative. It's just as important to **recognize the positive points,** so that the person feels valued and motivated. Starting by pointing out what has been done well helps establish a framework of trust before suggesting areas for improvement.

The benefits of constructive feedback

Constructive feedback, when well formulated, offers many benefits, both for individual development and for improving collective performance.

1. **Promotes professional development**: By receiving clear feedback on their actions, people can identify their strengths and areas for improvement. This encourages learning and development, while reinforcing motivation to progress.

2. **Reinforces trust and collaboration**: Feedback given in a respectful manner helps to establish a climate of trust and open dialogue. People who feel listened to and supported in their progress are more inclined to collaborate constructively with their colleagues.

3. **Correct mistakes quickly**: Constructive feedback helps to correct mistakes or inappropriate behavior before they

take root. Addressing a problem quickly and in a caring way can prevent it from escalating.

4. **Encourages good practice**: Giving positive feedback reinforces good behavior and encourages employees to continue in the same direction. This helps to establish a culture of recognition and appreciation of efforts within the team.

Active listening and constructive feedback

Effective feedback relies heavily on active listening. Before giving feedback, it's important to listen to the person, to understand their perspectives and feelings. This allows you to contextualize the feedback, avoid misunderstandings and adapt your message to the other person's reality. Similarly, when receiving feedback, active listening is essential to fully understand the points raised and identify areas for improvement.

By combining these two skills, we create a respectful and productive environment where everyone feels heard, valued and supported in their personal and professional development.

Conclusion

- **Final thoughts on the role of the cardiac orderly**
  - Importance of commitment and passion for the job

Commitment and passion for the job are essential elements that transcend the simple execution of daily tasks to instill real meaning and depth into the work. In healthcare professions such as nursing assistants, commitment and passion are not only appreciated qualities, but also values that are essential to the quality of care and well-being of patients. These two motivating forces give meaning to every professional gesture, transforming sometimes repetitive or trying tasks into acts imbued with compassion, dedication and responsibility. They are also essential drivers of resilience in the face of everyday difficulties and challenges.

Commitment: a pillar of quality care

Commitment to the profession means making a personal investment that goes beyond simply carrying out tasks. It's a commitment not only to one's own role, but above all to patients, colleagues and the care system as a whole. A committed caregiver is someone who does his or her utmost to give the best of themselves, at all times, considering each patient as a unique individual with specific needs.

In the context of care, commitment manifests itself in several ways:

1. **Assuming responsibility**: A committed caregiver takes his or her responsibilities to heart. They ensure that care protocols are rigorously followed, and that they anticipate patients' needs, even when they are not explicitly expressed. This commitment guarantees comprehensive, high-quality care. For example, a caregiver who cares about a patient's pain won't just follow medical instructions; he or she will also make sure that the patient feels listened to and understood, and will actively monitor any signs of deterioration.

2. **Taking initiative**: Commitment often goes hand in hand with **initiative**. A committed caregiver doesn't just wait to be told what to do; he or she makes informed decisions in the best interests of patients. For example, by anticipating a possible complication in a patient, they can alert the care team before the situation worsens.

3. **Involvement in patient relations**: Commitment to the nursing profession is not limited to technical gestures. It also means establishing a human relationship with patients, being attentive to their emotions and anxieties, and supporting them with empathy. A committed caregiver listens, reassures and accompanies patients on their healing journey, offering not only care, but also a comforting presence.

4. **Effective collaboration**: Commitment also means giving your best as part of the care team. A committed caregiver works collaboratively with other team members, sharing observations, listening to others, and proposing ideas to improve care. This investment in team spirit helps create a more harmonious working environment, where everyone feels supported.

Passion: a driving force in the face of challenges

Passion for the job is another essential ingredient that fuels commitment. It enables us to transcend the difficulties of everyday life, to face challenges with determination and to find meaning in the efforts we make. Passion for the nursing profession is above all a deep love of caring for others, a sincere desire to help, to relieve, and to make a difference in patients' lives.

1. **Finding meaning in every gesture**: Passion enables us to perceive every professional gesture not as a simple obligation, but as a meaningful act. Whether it's helping a patient get out of bed, providing hygiene care or

reassuring him or her after an operation, these gestures take on another dimension when passion drives the caregiver. It transforms the ordinary into an act of kindness and care. Giving meaning to every action boosts motivation and makes every working day more rewarding.

2. **Resisting burnout**: Working in the healthcare sector is often physically and psychologically demanding. Contact with illness, pain and sometimes death can take its toll on morale. This is where passion for the job becomes an essential driving force. It provides the extra energy needed to keep going, even in the most difficult of times. A passionate caregiver finds comfort in the idea that he or she is contributing, day after day, to improving the lives of others, which gives him or her the strength to overcome moments of fatigue or discouragement.

3. **Innovate and improve**: Passion also drives a constant desire to improve. A passionate caregiver is not satisfied with the status quo. They seek to develop their skills, learn new techniques and keep abreast of developments in the care field. This constant quest for personal and professional improvement is driven by a sincere desire to give patients the very best. For example, a passionate caregiver may take further training courses to acquire new skills, or suggest improvements to care protocols.

4. **Inspiring others**: Passion is contagious. When a caregiver is passionate about their profession, it shows in their attitude, enthusiasm and energy. This dynamism can inspire colleagues to get more involved and share the same passion for care. A team where passion is shared is a more cohesive, more motivated team, and therefore a more effective one.

The impact of commitment and passion on patients

The commitment and passion of caregivers have a direct and profound impact on the quality of care perceived by patients. A patient who feels that his or her caregiver is invested, attentive and passionate about his or her work will feel more confident and secure, and will be more inclined to follow medical recommendations.

1. **Creates a climate of trust**: A patient who perceives the commitment and passion of his caregiver will naturally feel better cared for. They will feel that their needs are a priority and that they are the center of attention. This trust enhances the care experience and promotes a more serene recovery.

2. **Reinforces adherence to care**: When a caregiver demonstrates genuine commitment and passion for his or her work, it's easier to convince the patient of the importance of following treatment or recommendations. The caregiver's authenticity and investment create a bond of trust, and the patient feels motivated to become actively involved in his or her own recovery.

3. **Improves patients' emotional well-being**: Caregiving is not just about treating physical symptoms; it's also about caring for patients' emotional well-being. A passionate and committed caregiver is able to perceive patients' anxieties or worries and reassure them with his or her presence, listening and kind words. This emotional support is just as important as medical care, helping patients to get through difficult times with greater serenity.

○ The future of the business: challenges and opportunities

The future of the nursing profession, and of healthcare professions in general, is taking shape against a backdrop of profound change in the medical sector. Between technological advances, an aging population and changing societal expectations, this profession is at the crossroads of numerous challenges and opportunities. The caregiver occupies a key position in the organization of care, and future developments, far from marginalizing this role, are enriching it and opening up new perspectives. Adapting to these changes requires the ability to reinvent oneself and integrate additional skills, while preserving the human values that are at the heart of the profession.

The challenges ahead

1. An ageing population

One of the major challenges facing the care sector is the **growing ageing of the population**. Medical advances, rising life expectancy and the ageing of the baby-boom generations are driving a considerable increase in the need for long-term care. For caregivers, this means an increased workload and the specific challenges of caring for elderly people, who are often multi-handicapped or suffering from chronic illnesses.

This population requires complex care, often focused on maintaining autonomy, managing chronic illnesses and preventing age-related complications (falls, malnutrition, bedsores). Faced with this situation, care assistants must not only master care techniques, but also develop an empathetic approach adapted to the psychological realities of the elderly, offering a sympathetic ear and taking into account the social dimension of care.

2. The evolution of chronic pathologies

Another major challenge is the **changing patient profile**. Chronic diseases such as diabetes, heart failure, respiratory diseases and obesity are on the rise. These pathologies require specific, often long-term care, with regular monitoring and daily management of treatments.

For caregivers, this means new skills, particularly in therapeutic education. Accompanying patients in the day-to-day management of their illnesses, helping them to understand and follow their treatments, and preventing complications become central tasks. This educational dimension of the caregiver's role represents a significant change, placing the carer not only in the role of executor, but also in that of **guide and companion to** the patient's health.

3. Staff shortages and workloads

The care sector has been experiencing **staff shortages** for several years in many countries, exacerbated by rising demand linked to ageing and the increase in chronic illnesses. Caregivers often find themselves understaffed, which can lead to **increased workloads**, a deterioration in the quality of working life, and increased **fatigue** or even burnout.

These difficult conditions represent a major challenge for the future of the profession. Caregivers will have to adapt to this pressure by developing skills in organization, time management and prioritizing care. Healthcare establishments will also have to rethink their human resources management policies to attract and retain professionals, while ensuring fairer working conditions that respect the well-being of caregivers.

4. The technological revolution

The medical sector, like many others, is in the midst of a **technological revolution**. The introduction of **new technologies** in healthcare, such as telemedicine tools, connected objects (blood pressure monitors, glucometers), medical monitoring software and assistance robots, is revolutionizing the day-to-day practice of caregivers.

For caregivers, this means acquiring new technological skills. While the integration of these tools into daily care practice opens up new possibilities, it can also create a distance with patients if these technologies are misunderstood or misused. The challenge is therefore to learn how to use these technologies without losing sight of the **human dimension** of care, which remains essential to the patient-caregiver relationship.

Opportunities for the future of the business

1. Developing skills and specializations

The future of the nursing profession offers numerous **opportunities** to **develop** and **enrich skills**. Evolving healthcare needs, such as chronic disease management, care of the elderly and palliative care, demand specific skills. Increasingly, care assistants will have the opportunity to **specialize** in fields such as gerontology, home care or rehabilitation, enabling them to meet new patient needs while enhancing their expertise.

Ongoing training programs will enable caregivers to keep up to date with medical and technological advances, and to acquire knowledge in a variety of fields, such as infection prevention, psychological support and therapeutic education. This increase in skills is an opportunity for caregivers to play a more active and recognized role in care teams.

2. Greater role in patient support

Care assistants are no longer seen as simply carrying out the care prescribed by nurses or doctors. Increasingly, their role as patient **companions** is becoming central. With the ageing of the population and the increase in chronic illnesses, care is no longer limited to technical gestures alone, but also includes overall support for the patient in his or her daily life, lifestyle choices and disease management.

This evolution represents an opportunity for caregivers to develop strong **interpersonal skills**, to play the role of privileged interlocutor with patients and their families, and to become genuine players in health promotion. This increased role in health education and prevention makes the nursing auxiliary a key element in the care process, and no longer simply a relay between the patient and the nurse or doctor.

3. New technologies for healthcare

If new technologies represent a challenge, they are also an **opportunity** to improve the quality of care and alleviate certain repetitive tasks. Assistive robots, for example, can be used to help patients move around or perform certain activities of daily living, enabling caregivers to concentrate more on human, relational care.

In addition, **telemedicine** tools enable more regular and precise monitoring of patients at home, particularly those with chronic illnesses. Caregivers can be trained to use these technologies to better monitor patients' vital signs, anticipate complications, and act more quickly when necessary. This will improve the quality of homecare and facilitate communication between patients, caregivers and medical teams.

4. Improved working conditions and greater recognition

Faced with the challenges posed by staff shortages and work overloads, many are calling for an **upgrading of care professions**, including that of nursing assistants. The future could see the emergence of healthcare policies that are more favorable to caregivers, with improved working conditions, higher salaries and greater recognition of their essential role.

Care assistants could thus benefit from **enhanced professional status**, with broader career development prospects, from specialization in a specific field to access to coordination positions within care structures. This increased recognition is not only an opportunity for caregivers to see their work valued, but also a lever for attracting new generations to the profession.

- **Incentives for future nurses' aides**
  - A final word: the caregiver's lasting impact on the health of cardiac patients

The caregiver's role with heart patients goes far beyond day-to-day care. It's part of a holistic support dynamic, where every gesture, every word and every attention contributes to the patient's **overall healing**, be it physical, emotional or psychological. The caregiver's lasting impact is felt on many levels, influencing the long-term health, well-being and even quality of life of cardiac patients. As a pillar of the care team, the caregiver plays a discreet but fundamental role in the success of care, creating an essential link between medical technique and the humanity of care.

Day-to-day support in a complex care pathway

Cardiac patients, whether hospitalized for an acute attack or regularly monitored for a chronic condition, face an often complex and sometimes distressing care pathway. The caregiver is present at every step of the way, offering a **reassuring presence** and constant support, day after day. They are the ones who help with daily tasks, monitor vital signs, and listen attentively to patients' concerns. By listening to their fears and pain, they play a key role in the overall care of the heart patient.

This daily presence enables the caregiver to **develop a relationship of trust** with the patient. This trust is essential, as it encourages patients to open up and share their doubts and symptoms, sometimes undetected by machines or medical tests. This enables us to react more quickly to early warning signs of cardiac complications. In this way, through their observations and ongoing dialogue with the patient, caregivers play an active role in preventing attacks and reducing complications.

A key player in post-operative care

The caregiver's impact doesn't stop at the hospital. After cardiac surgery, such as bypass or stenting, the patient's rehabilitation depends not only on technical care, but also on moral and physical support. Caregivers are often the ones who encourage patients to **gradually regain their autonomy**, helping them to get up, walk and regain self-confidence after a period of vulnerability. This support is fundamental to speeding up recovery.

What's more, **post-operative monitoring** by the nursing auxiliary is crucial to the early detection of any signs of complication, such as abnormal pain or unusual reactions. Their vigilance, combined with their in-depth knowledge of the patient, enables them to **react quickly**, guaranteeing better recovery and reducing the risk of readmission.

Essential emotional support

Beyond physical care, the caregiver plays an irreplaceable role in the **emotional support** of heart patients. Often faced with fear, anxiety and sometimes depression in the face of their illness, these patients need more than medical treatment. They need compassion, reassurance and the assurance that someone really cares about their well-being. The caregiver, by virtue of his or her proximity to patients, is the one who offers this human dimension to care.

This **empathy** is an essential factor in improving cardiac patients' quality of life. By taking the time to listen to their fears, reassure them about the healing process, and offer encouragement, the caregiver helps to **reduce their stress**, which is crucial in the management of heart disease. Studies show that stress management and psychological well-being have a direct impact on heart health, notably by reducing the risk of further attacks. In this way, the caregiver not only contributes to immediate recovery, but also to the **long-term prevention of** heart complications.

An educator for day-to-day management

One of the caregiver's most significant lasting impacts is his or her role as **educator**. After hospitalization or surgery, heart patients often need to adapt their lifestyle to avoid relapse. This involves modifying their diet, monitoring their blood pressure, incorporating appropriate physical activity and taking regular medication. The caregiver plays a key role in this transitional phase, explaining to patients the gestures to adopt, the signs to watch out for, and providing practical advice on how to better manage their day-to-day health.

This support is crucial to ensuring patients' **compliance with** their **treatment**, i.e. their ability to follow prescribed regimens correctly. By ensuring that patients understand what is at stake in their treatment, the caregiver helps to **reduce the risk of relapse**, and promotes better management at home. Thanks to these educational interactions, the caregiver's impact extends well beyond the hospital, having a lasting influence on the way patients manage their health in the long term.

A cornerstone of teamwork

Finally, the nursing auxiliary occupies a central position within the care team. They act as an **essential link** between nurses, doctors and other healthcare professionals. His or her position enables him or her to share valuable observations on the patient's condition, to quickly signal subtle changes in his or her state of health, and to **coordinate care** seamlessly. This **inter-professional collaboration** is crucial to ensuring comprehensive care, where each member of the team contributes his or her expertise, but where the caregiver remains a pillar of continuity of care.

By participating in this collective dynamic, the nursing auxiliary contributes not only to the immediate quality of care, but also to its **long-term effectiveness**, by ensuring that each patient benefits from coherent care adapted to his or her specific needs.